Recent Advances in

Surgery
32

Edited by

Irving Taylor MD ChM FRCS FMedSci FRCPS(Glas) FHEA
Vice-Dean and Director of Clinical Studies
Professor of Surgery, Royal Free and University College London Medical
School, University College London, London, UK

Colin D. Johnson MChir FRCS
Reader and Consultant Surgeon, University Surgical Unit, Southampton
General Hospital, Southampton, UK

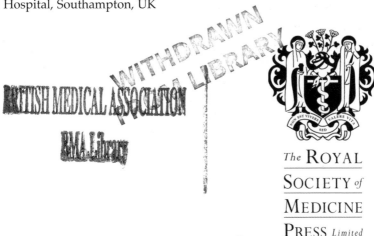

The ROYAL
SOCIETY *of*
MEDICINE
PRESS *Limited*

Published by the Royal Society of Medicine Press Ltd
1 Wimpole Street, London W1G 0AE, UK
Tel: +44 (0)20 7290 2921
Fax: +44 (0)20 7290 2929
Email: publishing@rsm.ac.uk
Website: www.rsmpress.co.uk

British Library Cataloguing in Publication Data
A catalogue record for this book is available from the British Library
ISBN 978–1–85315–874–2

Distribution in Europe and Rest of World:

Marston Book Services Ltd
PO Box 269, Abingdon
Oxon OX14 4YN, UK
Tel: +44 (0)1235 465500
Fax: +44 (0)1235 465555
Email: direct.order@marston.co.uk

Distribution in the USA and Canada:

Royal Society of Medicine Press Ltd
c/o BookMasters Inc
30 Amberwood Parkway
Ashland, OH 44805, USA
Tel: +1 800 247 6553/+1 800 266 5564
Fax: +1 419 281 6883
Email: order@bookmasters.com

Distribution in Australia and New Zealand:

Elsevier Australia
30-52 Smidmore Street
Marrickville NSW 2204, Australia
Tel: +61 2 9517 8999
Fax: +61 2 9517 2249
Email: service@elsevier.com.au

Editorial services and typesetting by GM & BA Haddock, Ford, Midlothian, UK

Printed in Great Britain by Bell & Bain, Glasgow, UK

Recent Advances in

Surgery
32

Recent Advances in Surgery 31
Edited by C. D. Johnson & I. Taylor

ISBN 978-1-85315-719-6

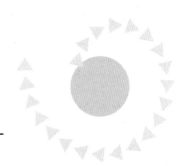

Contents

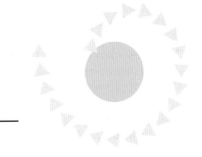

Contributors

Safa Al-Shamma MBChB MRCP
Specialist Registrar in Gastroenterology, Department of Medicine, Royal
Liverpool University Hospital, Royal Liverpool and Broadgreen University
Hospitals NHS Trust, Liverpool, UK

Shirish G. Ambekar MBBS MS MCh DMS FRCSEd(CTh)
Department of Cardiothoracic Surgery, St Bartholomew's Hospital, London, UK

Tan Arulampalam MD FRCS
Consultant Laparoscopic Surgeon and Service Director, The ICENI Centre,
Colchester General Hospital, Colchester, UK

James P. Byrne BSc MBChB MD FRCS
Consultant General and Upper Gastrointestinal Surgeon, Southampton General
Hospital, Southampton, UK

Arun Chaturvedi MS MAMS
Professor and Head, Department of Surgical Oncology, King George's Medical
University, Lucknow, India

Sarah Cheslyn-Curtis MBBS MS FRCS(Eng) FRCS(Gen)
Consultant Pancreatobiliary and General Paediatric Surgeon, Luton and
Dunstable Hospital, Luton, UK and Royal Free Hospital, London, UK

Michael Douek MBChB MD FRCS FRCS(Gen)
Reader in Surgery, Department of Research Oncology, Division of Cancer Studies,
King's College London, Guy's Hospital, London, UK

Mark A. Fox MBChB MRCP
Specialist Registrar in Gastroenterology, Department of Medicine, Royal
Liverpool University Hospital, Royal Liverpool and Broadgreen University
Hospitals NHS Trust, Liverpool, UK

Joanna Franks MBBS(Hons) BSc(Hons) MRCS MSc
Specialist Registrar in General Surgery, Division of Surgery and Interventional
Science, University College London, London, UK

Robert B. Galland MD FRCS
Consultant Surgeon, Department of Vascular Surgery, Royal Berkshire Hospital,
Reading, UK

Bawantha Gamage MS MRCS
Laparoscopic Fellow, The ICENI Centre, Colchester General Hospital, Colchester,
UK

Jonathan Hyde BSc MD FRCS
Consultant Cardiothoracic Surgeon, Sussex Cardiac Centre, Royal Sussex County Hospital, Brighton, UK

Atique Imam FRCS FRCR
Specialist Registrar in Radiology, Department of Radiology, John Radcliffe Hospital, Headington, Oxford, UK

Jan Jansen FRCS
Consultant Surgeon, Department of Surgery, Aberdeen Royal Infirmary, Aberdeen, UK

Colin D. Johnson MChir FRCS
Reader in Surgery and Consultant Surgeon, University Surgical Unit, Southampton General Hospital, Southampton, UK

Vasu Karri BSc(Hons) MRCS MSc
Specialist Registrar in Plastic Surgery, Melanoma Unit, Department of Plastic & Reconstructive Surgery, St George's Hospital NHS Trust, London, UK

Christopher Khoo FRCS
Consultant Plastic Surgeon, The Bridge Clinic, Maidenhead, Berkshire, UK

Kulvinder S. Lall MBBS FRCS(CTh)
Consultant Cardiothoracic Surgeon, St Bartholomew's Hospital, London, UK

Michael Lewis BSc MD FRCS
Consultant Cardiothoracic Surgeon, Sussex Cardiac Centre, Royal Sussex County Hospital, Brighton, UK

Malcolm A. Loudon MD FRCSEd(Gen)
Consultant Surgeon, Department of Surgery, Aberdeen Royal Infirmary, Aberdeen, UK

David Mahon MBChB MD FRCS(Gen)
Consultant Upper GI and Bariatric Surgeon, Musgrove Park NHS Trust, Taunton, UK

Peter McCulloch MBChB MA MD FRCS(Ed) FRCS(Glasg)
Clinical Reader in Surgery, Nuffield Department of Surgery, University of Oxford, John Radcliffe Hospital, Oxford, UK

Sanjeev Misra MS MCh FRCS FICS MAMS
Professor, Department of Surgical Oncology, King George's Medical University, Lucknow, India

Andrew R. Moore MBChB MRCP
Specialist Registrar in Gastroenterology, Department of Medicine, Royal Liverpool University Hospital, Royal Liverpool and Broadgreen University Hospitals NHS Trust, Liverpool, UK

John Morlese BSc FRCR
Consultant Radiologist, Department of Radiology, Leicester Royal Infirmary, Leicester, UK

Anthony I. Morris MSc MD FRCP
Honorary Professor in Gastroenterology at Liverpool and John Moores Universities, Department of Medicine, Royal Liverpool University Hospital, Royal Liverpool and Broadgreen University Hospitals NHS Trust, Liverpool, UK

Christopher Munsch ChM FRCS
Consultant Cardiothoracic Surgeon, Leeds General Infirmary, Leeds, UK

Raghu Ram Pillarisetti MS FRCS(Ed) FRCS(Glasg) FRCS(Irel)
Director and Consultant Oncoplastic Breast Surgeon, KIMS-Ushalakshmi Centre
for Breast Diseases, Krishna Institute of Medical Sciences (KIMS), Hyderabad,
India

Barry Powell MCh MA FRCS(Ed) FRCSE
Reader in Plastic Surgery, National Clinical Advisor in Skin Cancer, Head of
Melanoma Service, Melanoma Unit, Department of Plastic & Reconstructive
Surgery, St George's Hospital NHS Trust, London, UK

Jonathan K. Pye MBBS LRCP MRCS
Consultant Surgeon, Department of Surgery, Wrexham Maelor Hospital,
Wrexham, UK

Guidubaldo Querci della Rovere MD FRCS
Consultant Breast Surgeon, The Royal Marsden NHS Trust, Sutton, Surrey, UK

Shahab Siddiqi BSc FRCS(Gen)
Colorectal Fellow, Department of Colorectal Surgery, Castle Hill Hospital,
Cottingham, East Yorkshire, UK

Irving Taylor MD ChM FMedSci FRCPS(Glas) FHEA
Professor of Surgery, Director of Medical Studies and Vice Dean UCL Medical
School, University College London, London, UK

Bubby Thava MA MRCS
Specialist Registrar, Department of Vascular Surgery, Royal Berkshire Hospital,
Reading, UK

Michael Douek

1

Recognition and management of patients with inherited risk of breast cancer

Breast cancer is the most frequent neoplasm in women with over 45,500 new cases per annum in the UK.[1] Most women with breast cancer do not have a relevant family history of the disease. After female gender, the greatest risk factor for breast cancer is increasing age so that 8 in 10 breast cancers are diagnosed in women aged 50 years and over. Some women will have a relative diagnosed with breast cancer over 50 years of age but this is unlikely to be relevant in terms of increasing their risk of breast cancer. Others will have a cluster of close family members on the same side of the family diagnosed with breast cancer or a relative diagnosed at an early age (< 40 years), which may well increase their life-time risk of breast cancer. It has been estimated that up to 27% of women may have an inherited predisposition to breast cancer.[2] However, only about 5% are attributable to recognised genetic mutations which carry a very substantial life-time risk (> 50%) of breast cancer.[3]

Key points 1 and 2

- Most women with breast cancer do not have a relevant family history of the disease.

- After female gender, increasing age is the greatest risk factor for breast cancer.

Women presenting with a family history of breast cancer or a known relative with a genetic mutation, may harbour considerable anxiety which should be managed sensitively. Most women initially present in primary care and should be referred to the breast clinic at a specialist centre where

Michael Douek MBChB MD FRCS FRCS(Gen)
Reader in Surgery, Department of Research Oncology, Division of Cancer Studies, King's College London, 3rd Floor Bermondsey Wing, Guy's Hospital, Great Maze Pond, London SE1 9RT, UK.
E-mail : michel.douek@kcl.ac.uk

Table 1 Hereditary syndromes associated with an increase in the life-time risk of breast cancer

Syndrome	Gene
Hereditary breast and ovarian cancer syndrome	BRCA1 and BRCA2
Li–Fraumeni	p53
Cowden's disease	PTEN
Peutz–Jeghers syndrome	STK11/LKB1
Ataxic-telangiectasia	ATM
Hereditary diffuse gastric syndrome	CDH1
Variant of Li–Fraumeni	CHEK2

assessment and care can be provided by a multidisciplinary team. An initial clinical assessment will allow recognition of women who fall into the high or very high risk groups who can then be referred on for genetic counselling and be considered for genetic testing. Those women who are know genetic carriers or who fall into the high-risk group, have a number of management options open to them to reduce their risk. In addition, there are specific issues to consider when treating known mutation carriers diagnosed with breast cancer.

HEREDITARY SYNDROMES

Most women with a known genetic predisposition have a mutation of one of two genes BRCA1 or BRCA2.[4] There are other genetic mutations associated with an increased life-time risk of breast cancer which are found within recognised syndromes (Table 1). The commonest and most important is the hereditary breast and ovarian cancer syndrome.

HEREDITARY BREAST AND OVARIAN CANCER SYNDROME

Hereditary breast and ovarian cancer syndrome, linked to mutations in BRCA1 and BRCA2, should be suspected in patients with multiple close relatives with breast cancer or ovarian cancer (diagnosed under 50 years of age), a relative with bilateral breast cancer or male relative with breast cancer. BRCA1 and BRCA2 genes are transmitted in an autosomal dominant fashion and thus can be inherited from the maternal or paternal side. BRCA1 has been linked to a range of cellular processes including DNA repair, transcriptional regulation and chromatin remodelling. BRCA2 is involved in DNA recombination and is also involved in DNA repair. Mutations of these genes are associated with a 36–85% life-time risk of breast cancer and 16–60% life-time risk of ovarian cancer.[5,6] The life-time risk of other cancers is also increased including

Key points 3 and 4
- Less than 5% of women with breast cancer carry a known genetic mutation.
- Up to 27% of women may have an inherited predisposition for breast cancer.

peritoneal, fallopian tube, prostate and pancreatic cancers. Male mutation carriers of BRCA1 and BRCA2 have an estimated 1.2% and 6.8% life-time risk of breast cancer, respectively.[7] Numerous mutations have been identified and specific founder mutations are more prevalent in certain ethnic populations including Ashkenazi Jewish, Norwegian, Dutch and Icelandic.[8] In the Ashkenazi Jewish population, three founder mutations (two in the BRCA1 and one in the BRCA2 genes) account for almost all mutations.

RISK ASSESSMENT

Obtaining a family history, in order to draw up a family tree, is the first step in risk assessment. Patients with a significant family history should be referred to a breast clinic or family history clinic for further assessment. The TRACE study (Trial of Genetic Assessment in Breast Cancer) demonstrated that psychological outcome following a surgical consultation at a breast clinic was similar to that of a surgical consultation with an additional consultation by a geneticist.[9]

In the UK, the life-time risk of breast cancer for women is approximately 11% or 1 in 9. The published guidelines for the UK Cancer Family Study Group[10] can be used to estimate familial risk. Several assessment tools and computer software are available to estimate an individual's life-time risk of breast cancer (e.g. Gail model, Claus tables, Tyrer-Cuzick) and also the likelihood of a deleterious BRCA mutation (e.g. BRCAPRO) taking into account epidemiological factors and family history. However, these models tend to underestimate risk in a family history setting and there is a poor correlation between different assessment tools.[11] It is also important to note that, in patients with a known genetic mutation, penetrance varies considerably in difference families and this is more difficult to account for.

Key point 5 and 6

- Women with a high life-time risk of breast cancer should be managed in a specialist unit.
- BRCA 1 and BRCA 2 are the commonest genetic mutations and predispose patients to cancer including breast, ovarian, fallopian tube, prostate, pancreatic and peritoneal.

Life-time risk can be estimated and classified into three broad categories (Table 2). Sauven et al.[12] and the UK National Institute for Health and Clinical Excellence (NICE)[11] have used this type of classification as an aid to

Table 2 Classification of life-time risk[11,12]

Risk group	Of population (%)	Life-time risk (%)	Relative life-time risk
Near population 'low'	97%	< 1:6 (17%)	< 2
Moderate	2%	≥ 1:6 (17%) to 1:4 (25%)	2–3
High	< 1%	> 1:4 (25%)	> 3

recommend which patients to refer to a secondary or tertiary centre, which to refer for genetic counselling, when to recommend genetic testing and which patients should be offered early screening or a risk-reducing strategy. In general terms, women with at least two first degree relatives diagnosed under the age of 40 years (or three under the age of 50 years), more than one relative with ovarian cancer with or without breast cancer, or a known gene carrier, fall into the high-risk category and should be referred for genetic counselling.

Key point 7

- Several assessment tools and computer software are available to estimate an individual's life-time risk of breast cancer (*e.g.* Gail model, Claus tables, Tyrer-Cuzick) and also the likelihood of a deleterious BRCA mutation (*e.g.* BRCAPRO).

GENETIC COUNSELLING AND TESTING

Genetic counselling should be undertaken within a cancer genetics clinic where appropriate counselling by specialists is available.[12] Patients at a moderate or high life-time risk, should be referred to a cancer genetics clinic.

GENETIC TESTING

Genetic testing is only recommended in patients who have a high risk of a BRCA mutation or a strong clinical suspicious of a specific syndrome. In the UK, genetic testing is recommended for patients with a life-time risk of breast cancer of 20% or over,[12] whereas in America, it is recommended with a life-time risk of breast cancer of 10% or over.[13,14] Genetic testing is not recommended in patients at a low risk of a BRCA mutation or the general population at present, outside clinical trials. This is because of the risk of falsely labelling patients as having a genetic predisposition which has potential ethical, legal, financial and social consequences.[6]

Genetic testing usually requires a patient to have a living affected relative (with breast or ovarian cancer) who will undertake genetic testing in order to identify a specific mutation (the diagnostic genetic test). If a BRCA mutation is identified, the patient can then be tested for this mutation (the predictive genetic test).[12] If the patient is found to be negative, this is a true negative and thus the patient does not carry the mutation and can be re-assured. The patient's life-time risk of breast cancer would be expected to be equal to, or less than, that of the general population. However, if a BRCA mutation is not

---

Key point 8

- Genetic testing is only recommended in patients who have a high risk of a BRCA mutation or a strong clinical suspicion of a specific syndrome.

found, this is not a clinically useful result since other undetected mutations of other genes, or other factors, could account for the patient's family history of breast cancer.

MANAGEMENT OPTIONS

Patients with a high life-time risk of breast cancer fall into one of three categories: (i) those with an identified genetic mutation; (ii) those with a strong family history but without an identifiable genetic mutation; and (iii) those with a strong family history who have not been, or could not be, tested. Several options are available with the intention of early diagnosis (screening) or reducing the life-time risk (risk-reducing). None of these are supported by evidence from randomised controlled trials with appropriate end-points (*e.g.* survival), specifically applicable to this patient population. However, there is some evidence to support intervention in this group of patients.

SCREENING

The purpose of screening is to detect breast cancers before they become palpable and, through early treatment, reduce mortality. Breast self-examination is sometimes recommended in addition to screening but two large population-based trials have not demonstrated any reduction in breast cancer mortality.[15–17] Furthermore, almost twice as many benign biopsies were performed in the screening group, suggesting a potential for increased morbidity with breast self-examination. Clinical breast examination alone has not been evaluated within a randomised controlled trial. However, in four of the nine randomised controlled trials of mammographic screening,[18,19] clinical breast examination was undertaken together with mammography suggesting some benefit.[18,20]

BRCA mutation carriers are also at risk of ovarian cancer. The are no randomised controlled trials demonstrating that ovarian cancer screening can reduce mortality. CA-125 and transvaginal ultrasound are in use and these should be undertaken within clinical trials or strict unit protocols.

The radiological options available for breast screening are mammography and breast magnetic resonance imaging (MRI) but neither is supported by randomised controlled trials specifically applicable to this patient population. Ultrasound has been shown to improve the detection of cancers when used as an adjunct to mammography in women with dense breasts; however, its role as a primary screening tool in younger women is not supported by randomised controlled trials.[21]

Mammography

Screening mammography has now been demonstrated to reduce mortality in women over the age of 50 years, but screening from the age of 40 years is still controversial. Screening mammography has been evaluated in nine large randomised trials with long follow-up.[18,19] Despite methodological criticisms of all the screening trials, a meta-analysis from Sweden estimated the reduction in breast cancer mortality to be 21%.[22] It has also been estimated that for every 2000 women screened for 10 years, only 1 women will have her life prolonged.[18]

Patients with a moderate or high life-time risk of breast cancer who are being considered for screening, tend to be in their thirties or forties. Breast cancer deaths as a proportion of all female deaths are higher for women in their forties and approximately one-third of the life years lost to breast cancer are from this group. However, mammographic screening in women below 50 years of age was not found to beneficial in adequately randomised trials.[18,19] Screening mammography in this age group is not advocated in the general UK population. The FH01 study was launched in the UK in 2003. It is a large, non-randomised, observational study recruiting 6000 women aged 40–44 years with a family history of breast cancer referred for mammographic screening. The authors hope to assess the impact of annual invitation to mammographic screening in women within the 40–49 years of age group with moderate-to-high life-time risk of breast cancer.[23] At present, mammographic screening in younger groups at familial risk is of unproven benefit and should only be undertaken within strict unit protocols or clinical trials.[12]

There is a potential harmful effect from the ionising radiation used in mammography and it has been suggested that since the BRCA1 and BRCA2 genes are involved with DNA repair, mammography could prove more harmful in mutation carriers.[24] However, this has not been demonstrated and radiation exposure has been decreasing with the introduction of digital mammography.[25]

Breast MRI

Contrast-enhanced MRI is a very sensitive test when compared to mammography but has a low specificity and has not been demonstrated to reduce breast cancer mortality in this or any other patient population. The greatest clinical utility of breast MRI is in women at high-risk and those with genetic predisposition. This was demonstrated in several trials including MARIBS, a prospective randomised controlled trial.[26] MRI is also useful for imaging younger patients with dense breasts. However, false-positive findings are well recognised and may require further diagnostic intervention. NICE has recently published an update on the management of familial breast cancer, recommending the use of breast MRI for screening women with an increased risk of breast cancer, according to their estimated 10-year risk.[27]

CHEMOPREVENTION

Tamoxifen has been known to reduce the risk of contralateral breast cancer for over 20 years.[28] This led to the hypothesis that tamoxifen could prevent breast cancer. An overview of all four trials concluded that tamoxifen reduces the risk of invasive breast cancer by 38% (95% CI, 28– 46%; $P < 0.0001$),[29] but this was not specifically demonstrated in mutation carriers. However, long-term tamoxifen use is associated with thrombo-embolic complications and significantly increases the risk of endometrial cancer. Its use should be restricted to patients at high risk of breast cancer and low risk of complications.[12] Although it should be discussed as an option, the optimal duration of treatment is also unknown. Trials to evaluate other agents such as Raloxifen and aromatase inhibitors, are currently underway. In the UK, the International Breast Cancer Intervention Study II (IBIS II) is currently underway comparing anastrazole to placebo in chemoprevention of high-risk post-menopausal women.[30]

RISK-REDUCING SURGERY

To reduce the life-time risk of breast and ovarian cancer, BRCA1 and BRCA2 carriers and high-risk patients can be offered risk-reducing surgery. There are no prospective, randomised, controlled trials to support this although some retrospective studies suggest a dramatic reduction in life-time risk. In addition, the risk of other cancers (*e.g.* prostate, peritoneal) is likely to be unaffected.

A paradox exists between the treatment of women who present with breast cancer and those who present without cancer but with a high life-time risk. The standard surgical treatment for most patients with operable breast cancer is breast-conserving surgery whereas for high-risk women, it is bilateral mastectomy. This is a major decision that requires time and a multidisciplinary approach.[11] Patients should have already been assessed by a clinical geneticist and should have an estimated life-time risk of breast cancer of 25–30%. They should have been provided with an assessment of their risk, presented in several ways so as to facilitate their understanding. All management options should have been considered and the patients should be fully informed about the type of surgical procedures and their complications. The timing of surgery is also complicated by psychosocial issues and some women may benefit from formal assessment.

Bilateral mastectomy

The aims of risk-reducing mastectomy are to reduce the incidence of breast cancer, reduce mortality and minimise the impact on cosmesis and quality of life. Risk-reducing mastectomy reduces the life-time risk of breast cancer in BRCA1 and BRCA 2 carriers by about 90%,[31,32] but does not remove the risk completely. If the nipple is preserved, it is estimated that about 10% of breast cancers arise centrally, deep to the nipple areola complex.[33] Patients should be informed of this and nipple excision recommended particularly in known BRCA1 or BRCA2 mutation carriers.[12]

There are several surgical approaches for risk-reducing mastectomy and primary breast reconstruction. This should be undertaken by a specialist surgeon within a specialist unit who has an interest in oncoplastic surgery or in conjunction with a specialist oncoplastic surgeon. The aim is to remove virtually all the breast tissue including the axillary tail, and provide the patient with a good cosmetic result. This often requires several separate procedures including nipple reconstruction. The surgical options include, bilateral subcutaneous mastectomy (preserving the skin envelope and nipple), bilateral skin-sparing mastectomy (preserving the skin envelope but removing the nipple) or total bilateral mastectomy. The reconstructive options include silicon implant reconstruction or autologous myocutaneous flaps (with or without a silicon implant). Autologous reconstruction is usually undertaken with a latissimus dorsi or free deep inferior epigastric (DIEP) flap.

Contralateral mastectomy

Many BRCA1 and BRCA2 mutation carriers are diagnosed after breast-conserving surgery for cancer. In this circumstance, a decision needs to be taken about the need for a risk-reducing completion mastectomy and contralateral mastectomy, with or without reconstruction. Following adjuvant radiotherapy, some women may have post-radiation change and this may increase the chance of complications on that side.

Bilateral oophorectomy

BRCA mutation carriers are also at a considerable risk of developing ovarian cancer. Bilateral salpingo-oophorectomy is usually undertaken in view of the increased risk of fallopian tube cancer as well. It is usually performed laparoscopically and is a much more acceptable operation to mutation carriers. The timing of surgery depends on an individual's perception of risk and whether or not they have completed their family.

Oophorectomy can reduce the life-time risk of ovarian cancer in BRCA carriers by about 90%. Pre-menopausal oophorectomy can also reduce the life-time risk of breast cancer by up to 50%.[34]

TREATMENT OF BREAST CANCER

Many high-risk women and BRCA mutation carriers are diagnosed after presenting with breast cancer. In this situation, there is limited time to consider bilateral mastectomy. Bilateral mastectomy at the time of presenting with breast cancer is more acceptable to women in North America than it is in Europe.[35]

Breast-conserving surgery and radiotherapy are feasible in mutation carriers but they are at an increased risk of developing second primaries, particularly in the contralateral breast.[36] Decisions on indication for sentinel node biopsy and need for systemic therapy are based on standard clinical and pathological factors.

CONCLUSIONS

Patients with a significant family history of breast cancer should be referred to a breast or family history clinic for assessment. Those patients with a moderate-to-high life-time risk should be referred to a specialist cancer genetics clinic for assessment and genetic counselling. This should include formal risk assessment and a discussion about the full range of risk-reducing measures. There is no prospective, randomised, controlled data supporting early screening or risk-reducing measures. Patients should, therefore, be encouraged to participate in existing clinical trials.

Key points for clinical practice

- Most women with breast cancer do not have a relevant family history of the disease.
- After female gender, increasing age is the greatest risk factor for breast cancer.
- Less than 5% of women with breast cancer carry a known genetic mutation.
- Up to 27% of women may have an inherited predisposition for breast cancer.

Key points for clinical practice (continued)

- Women with a high life-time risk of breast cancer should be managed in a specialist unit.

- BRCA 1 and BRCA 2 are the commonest genetic mutations and predispose patients to cancer including breast, ovarian, fallopian tube, prostate, pancreatic and peritoneal.

- Several assessment tools and computer software are available to estimate an individual's life-time risk of breast cancer (*e.g.* Gail model, Claus tables, Tyrer-Cuzick) and also the likelihood of a deleterious BRCA mutation (*e.g.* BRCAPRO).

- Genetic testing is only recommended in patients who have a high risk of a BRCA mutation or a strong clinical suspicion of a specific syndrome.

References

1. Office for National Statistics. *Cancer statistics – registrations. Registrations of cancer diagnosed in 2005, England.* Series MB1 no. 36. Newport: Office for National Statistics, 2008.
2. Peto J, Mack TM. High constant incidence in twins and other relatives of women with breast cancer. *Nat Genet* 2000; **26**: 411–414.
3. Ford D, Easton DF, Sratton M *et al.* Genetic heterogeneity and penetrance analysis of the BRCA1 and BRCA2 genes in breast cancer families. The Breast Cancer Linkage Consortium. *Am J Hum Genet* 1998; **62**: 676–689.
4. Robson M, Offit K. Clinical practice. Management of an inherited predisposition to breast cancer. *N Engl J Med* 2007; **357**: 154–162.
5. Levy-Lahad E, Friedman E. Cancer risks among BRCA1 and BRCA2 mutation carriers. *Br J Cancer* 2007; **96**: 11–15.
6. Jatoi I, Anderson WF. Management of women who have a genetic predisposition for breast cancer. *Surg Clin North Am* 2008; **88**: 845–861.
7. Tai YC, Domchek S, Parmigiani G, Chen S. Breast cancer risk among male BRCA1 and BRCA2 mutation carriers. *J Natl Cancer Inst* 2007; **99**: 1811–1814.
8. Ferla R, Calo V, Cascio S *et al.* Founder mutations in BRCA1 and BRCA2 genes. *Ann Oncol* 2007; (**18 Suppl 6**): vi93–vi98.
9. Brain K, Gray J, Norman P *et al.* Randomized trial of a specialist genetic assessment service for familial breast cancer. *J Natl Cancer Inst* 2000; **92**: 1345–1351.
10. Eccles DM, Evans DG, Mackay J. Guidelines for a genetic risk based approach to advising women with a family history of breast cancer. UK Cancer Family Study Group (UKCFSG). *J Med Genet* 2000; **37**: 203–209.
11. National Institute for Health and Clinical Excellence. *Clinical guidelines for the classification and care of women at risk of familial breast cancer in primary, secondary and tertiary care.* Clinical Guideline 14. London: NICE, 2004.
12. Sauven P, Association of Breast Surgery Family History Guidelines Panel. Guidelines for the management of women at increased familial risk of breast cancer. *Eur J Cancer* 2004; **40**: 653–665.
13. American Society of Clinical Oncology policy statement update: genetic testing for cancer susceptibility. *J Clin Oncol* 2003; **21**: 2397–2406.
14. Berliner JL, Fay AM. Risk assessment and genetic counseling for hereditary breast and ovarian cancer: recommendations of the National Society of Genetic Counselors. *J Genet Counsel* 2007; **16**: 241–260.
15. Kosters JP, Gotzsche PC. Regular self-examination or clinical examination for early

detection of breast cancer. *Cochrane Database Syst Rev* 2003; CD003373.

16. Semiglazov VF, Manilhas AG, Moiseenko VM *et al.* [Results of a prospective randomized investigation [Russia (St Petersburg)/WHO] to evaluate the significance of self-examination for the early detection of breast cancer]. *Vopr Onkol* 2003; **49**: 434–441.

17. Thomas DB, Gao DL, Ray RM *et al.* Randomized trial of breast self-examination in Shanghai: final results. *J Natl Cancer Inst* 2002; **94**: 1445–1457.

18. Gotzche PC, Nielsen M. Screening for breast cancer with mammography. *Cochrane Database Syst Rev* 2006; CD001877.

19. Moss SM, Cuckle H, Evans A *et al.* Effect of mammographic screening from age 40 years on breast cancer mortality at 10 years' follow-up: a randomised controlled trial. *Lancet* 2006; **368**: 2053–2060.

20. Miller AB, To T, Baines CJ, Wall C. Canadian National Breast Screening Study-2: 13-year results of a randomized trial in women aged 50-59 years. *J Natl Cancer Inst* 2000; **92**: 1490–1499.

21. Irwig L, Houssami N, van Vliet C. New technologies in screening for breast cancer: a systematic review of their accuracy. *Br J Cancer* 2004; **90**: 2118–2122.

22. Nystrom L, Andersson I, Bjurstam N *et al.* Long-term effects of mammography screening: updated overview of the Swedish randomised trials. *Lancet* 2002; **359**: 909–919.

23. The FH01 Management Committee, Steering Committee and Collaborators. The challenge of evaluating annual mammography screening for young women with a family history of breast cancer. *J Med Screen* 2006; **13**: 177–182.

24. Pisano ED, Gasonis CG, Hendrik E *et al.* Diagnostic performance of digital versus film mammography for breast-cancer screening. *N Engl J Med* 2005; **353**: 1773–1783.

25. Leach MO, Boggis CR, Dixon AK *et al.* Screening with magnetic resonance imaging and mammography of a UK population at high familial risk of breast cancer: a prospective multicentre cohort study (MARIBS). *Lancet* 2005; **365**: 1769–1778.

26. National Institute for Health and Clinical Excellence. *Familial breast cancer: the classification and care of women at risk of familial breast cancer in primary, secondary and tertiary care (partial update of CG14).* Reference CG041. London: NICE, 2006.

27. Cuzick J, Baum M. Tamoxifen and contralateral breast cancer. *Lancet* 1985; **2**: 282.

28. Cuzick J, Powles T, Veronesi U *et al.* Overview of the main outcomes in breast-cancer prevention trials. *Lancet* 2003; **361**: 296–300.

29. Cuzick J. IBIS II: a breast cancer prevention trial in postmenopausal women using the aromatase inhibitor Anastrozole. *Expert Rev Anticancer Ther* 2008; **8**: 1377–1385.

30. Meijers-Heijboer H, van Geel B, van Putten WLJ *et al.* Breast cancer after prophylactic bilateral mastectomy in women with a BRCA1 or BRCA2 mutation. *N Engl J Med* 2001; **345**: 159–164.

31. Hartmann LC, Sellers TA, Schaid DJ *et al.* Efficacy of bilateral prophylactic mastectomy in BRCA1 and BRCA2 gene mutation carriers. *J Natl Cancer Inst* 2001; **93**: 1633–1637.

32. Lagios MD, Gates EA, Westdahl PR, Richards V, Alpert BS. A guide to the frequency of nipple involvement in breast cancer. A study of 149 consecutive mastectomies using a serial subgross and correlated radiographic technique. *Am J Surg* 1979; **138**: 135–142.

33. Rebbeck TR, Lynch HT, Neuhausen SL *et al.* Prophylactic oophorectomy in carriers of BRCA1 or BRCA2 mutations. *N Engl J Med* 2002; **346**: 1616–1622.

34. Metcalfe KA, Lubinski J, Ghadirian P *et al.* Predictors of contralateral prophylactic mastectomy in women with a BRCA1 or BRCA2 mutation: the Hereditary Breast Cancer Clinical Study Group. *J Clin Oncol* 2008; **26**: 1093–1097.

35. Domchek SM, Armstrong K, Weber BL. Clinical management of BRCA1 and BRCA2 mutation carriers. *Nat Clin Pract Oncol* 2006; **3**: 2–3.

Raghu Ram Pillarisetti
Guidubaldo Querci della Rovere

2

Oncoplastic breast surgery

Breast surgery is now a recognised subspecialty of general surgery with structured training for designated 'breast surgeons'. Over recent years, breast cancer care has been enhanced by the emergence of specialist breast surgeons with training in oncoplastic surgical skills – the oncoplastic breast surgeon.[1-3]

Oncoplastic breast surgery is one of the most interesting and challenging new developments of the last 20 years. The aims of oncoplastic surgery are wide local excision of the cancer coupled with partial reconstruction of the defect to achieve a cosmetically acceptable result. Avoidance of mastectomy and consequent reduction of psychological morbidity are the principal goals in the development of various oncoplastic techniques. The focus of this chapter is to highlight the principles governing the art and science of oncoplastic breast-conserving surgery.

Key points 1 and 2

- Over recent years, breast cancer care has been enhanced by the emergence of the specialist breast surgeon with training in oncoplastic surgical skills – the oncoplastic breast surgeon.

- The aims of oncoplastic surgery are wide local excision of the cancer coupled with partial reconstruction of the defect to achieve a cosmetically good result. Avoidance of mastectomy and consequent reduction of psychological morbidity are the principal goals in the development of various oncoplastic techniques.

Raghu Ram Pillarisetti MS FRCS(Ed) FRCS(Glasg) FRCS(Irel) (for correspondence)
Director and Consultant Oncoplastic Breast Surgeon, KIMS-Ushalakshmi Centre for Breast Diseases,
Krishna Institute of Medical Sciences (KIMS), Hyderabad, India.
E-mail: p.raghuram@hotmail.com

Guidubaldo Querci della Rovere MD FRCS
Consultant Breast Surgeon, The Royal Marsden NHS Trust, Downs Road, Sutton, Surrey SM2 5PT, UK

THE BASICS

Randomised, controlled trials (RCTs) over the past two decades have now established that mastectomy and breast-conserving surgery are equivalent in terms of survival,[4,5] provided local recurrence rates after breast conservation surgery are kept at about 1% per annum.[6]

Oncoplastic surgery should not be either identified or confused with breast reconstructive surgery after mastectomy. Whereas it is possible for a breast surgeon to perform a mastectomy and then allow the plastic surgeon to carry out the reconstruction, this is not feasible in oncoplastic breast conservative surgery, as it requires knowledge both of oncological and plastic surgery combined in one person for a good oncological and cosmetic outcome.

The concept of the oncoplastic breast surgeon is a new one for which formal training is still not fully developed. The difficulty lies in the fact that it requires the combination of knowledge in three different specialties – surgical oncology, plastic surgery and breast radiology.

An oncoplastic breast surgeon has to address three questions before undertaking oncoplastic, breast-conserving surgery:

1. *Can the cancer be removed with a simple wide local excision and a good cosmetic result?*

2. *If not, would an oncoplastic technique either at the outset or after neo-adjuvant systemic treatment reduce the risk of positive margins requiring a subsequent mastectomy?*

3. *Are the chances of achieving clear margins so small that breast conservation might not be advisable (although the patient might be willing to take a small chance)?*

The answer to these questions is often not easy and requires considerable knowledge and experience not only in oncological and oncoplastic surgery, but also, more importantly, in radiological assessment of the breast. A careful evaluation of the extent of disease by mammographic, ultrasonographic and sometimes magnetic resonance imaging (MRI) techniques, its nearness to the nipple and the distribution of the cancer in either radial or circumferential manner are all essential to the planning and the eventual success of the procedure.

Contrary to popular belief a few years ago, we now know that in some cases ipsilateral breast cancer local recurrence can be a determinant cause of death from the disease and, therefore, every attempt must be made to reduce the risk of local recurrence.[6]

The oncoplastic surgical techniques described below avoid a mastectomy in carefully selected patients, achieve wider margins of excision and, therefore, reduce the risk of local recurrence and produce good cosmetic results.

Key point 3

• Oncoplastic surgery should not be confused with breast reconstructive surgery after mastectomy. The oncoplastic breast surgeon requires the combination of knowledge in thee different specialties: – surgical oncology, plastic surgery and breast radiology.

CRITERIA FOR BREAST-CONSERVING SURGERY

The criteria for breast conserving surgery are relative. Contrary to traditional teaching, breast-conserving surgery is feasible every time it is judged possible to achieve complete surgical excision with good cosmesis. The size of the tumour relative to the breast volume is the deciding factor in determining the suitability of breast conserving surgery. It may even be suitable for women with large breasts in whom the tumour is up to 5 cm in size or even multifocal tumours confined to the same quadrant and when large operable tumours have been down-staged by neo-adjuvant chemotherapy.[7] The use of plastic surgical techniques not only ensures good cosmetic outcome, but also allows the cancer surgeon to remove the tumour with a greater volume of surrounding tissue, thus extending the boundaries of breast-conserving surgery.

PLANNING AND CHOICE OF INCISION

Poor planning in breast-conserving surgery can result in unacceptable deformity. Bad cosmetic outcome following breast-conserving surgery occurs due to combination of factors such as wrongly placed incision, poor surgical technique resulting in local glandular defect and scar contracture.

The choice of incision is crucial. Radial incisions in the lower part of the breast and circumlinear incisions in the upper half result in least visible scars. The incisions for dealing with lesions in the upper and outer quadrant of the breast should ideally be separate from the axillary incision to prevent scar contracture.[8]

Good cosmetic outcome can be obtained if deeper glandular tissue is approximated to obliterate glandular defect. After excision of the lesion, the breast tissue must be mobilised both at the level of the pectoral fascia and the subcutaneous plane to allow tension-free approximation of tissues.

Based on the clock position of the lesion in the left breast, the suggested incisions would be as follows:[8,9]

12 o'clock	*Circumareolar (with or without medial/lateral extensions), circumferential or round block technique (Figs 1–4).*
1–4 o'clock	*Radial or lateral mammoplasty; if concomitant axillary dissection is required, the axillary incision should be on the lower skin crease of the axilla and border of the pectoralis major muscle. For larger cancers, the two incisions can be joined together to allow better mobilisation and reconstruction of the breast parenchyma.*
5 and 6 o'clock	*Slightly 'comma'-shaped, superior pedicle reduction or glandular rotation (Fig. 5).*
7 and 8 o'clock	*Radial, glandular rotation, thoraco-epigastric flap or breast reduction (superior [Figs 6–9] or inferior [Figs 10–14] pedicle).*
9 o'clock	*Radial or round block technique.*
10 and 11 o'clock	*Circumferential or round block technique.*
Retro-areolar (central)	*Grisotti advancement rotation flap (Figs 15–19).*

Key points 4–6

- Proper patient selection and careful planning after proper radio-logical and clinical assessment are the two essential prerequisites before undertaking oncoplastic, breast-conserving surgery.

- Bad cosmetic outcome following breast-conserving surgery occurs due to a combination of factors such as wrongly placed incision, poor surgical technique resulting in local glandular defect and scar contracture.

- Good cosmetic outcome can be obtained if deeper glandular tissue is approximated to obliterate glandular defect. After excision of the lesion, the breast tissue must be mobilised at the level of the pectoral fascia and the subcutaneous plane to allow tension-free approximation of tissues.

VOLUME DISPLACEMENT AND REPLACEMENT

Oncoplastic surgery involves both volume displacement and volume replacement techniques. However, volume displacement is more common in the context of breast-conserving surgery, which is done at the same sitting rather than as delayed procedure. When the tumour is large in a relatively large breast, reduction mammoplasty (breast-reducing surgery) can be fashioned using the nipple areola pedicle based either superiorly or inferiorly.

VOLUME DISPLACEMENT TECHNIQUES

The commonly used volume displacement procedures are:[8,9]

1. **Superior pedicle breast reduction** for cancers in the lower part of the breast Figs 6–9.

2. **Inferior pedicle breast** reduction for cancers above the nipple or in the lower medial or lateral quadrants (Figs 10–14).

3. **Grisotti advancement rotation flap** for small tumours in the central quadrant of the breast (retro-areolar region) (Figs 15–19).

4. **Round block technique** for cancers in the upper and inner quadrant of the breast or in the 12 o'clock position(Figs 1–4).

5. **Local glandular flaps**: glandular rotation for tumours in the lower inner quadrant and 6 o'clock position (Fig. 21). Thoraco-epigastric flap for tumours in the lower inner quadrants (Fig. 20).

6. **Lateral mammoplasty** for tumours in the upper outer quadrants (but not in the 12 o'clock position in which case a round block is preferable; Fig. 22).

7. **Horizontal mammoplasty** for tumours above the level of the nipple but at least 18–20 cm below the clavicle Figs 23 and 24).

Key points 7–9

- Oncoplastic surgery involves both volume displacement and volume replacement techniques. The indications for cosmetically acceptable breast-conserving surgery can be safely extended to tumours involving all the quadrants of the breast, thus expanding the armamentarium of oncoplastic surgery.

- The use of plastic surgical techniques not only ensures good cosmetic outcome, but also allows the cancer surgeon to remove the tumour with greater volume of surrounding tissue, thus extending the boundaries of breast-conserving surgery.

- The need for adjustment of contralateral breast should also be anticipated at the time of planning breast-conserving surgery. The primary aim is to correct any asymmetry between the operated breast and contralateral one. Contralateral oncoplastic surgery can be done either at the same time as breast cancer surgery or as a delayed setting.

VOLUME REPLACEMENT TECHNIQUES

Extensive resection in the breast could be replaced with volume (volume replacement procedure). Mini latisimus dorsi flap is the commonly used flap to cover these defects. Patients should be counselled about an additional scar in the donor area, differences of colour and feel of the latisimus dorsi flap compared to the normal breast and that the option of latisimus dorsi flap reconstruction will not be available in the event of the patient developing a recurrence requiring a completion mastectomy.[8]

ONCOPLASTIC SURGERY AFTER RADIOTHERAPY

Oncoplastic breast surgery following radiotherapy is more complex. The breast tissue is less robust and less vascular; hence, surgery is associated with potential complications. Contralateral breast reduction should be considered as an option to deal with breast asymmetry following radiotherapy and surgery should be avoided on the irradiated breast. Should there be gross deformity following radiotherapy to the breast, volume replacement technique, such as mini latissimus dorsi flap should be employed to correct the defect.[8] Myocutaneous flap, like the latisimus dorsi flap is best suited in this scenario as it brings fresh blood supply to the area.

Key point 10

- Extensive resection in the breast could be replaced with volume (volume replacement procedure). The mini latissimus dorsi flap is commonly used to cover these defects. The clinician and the patient must, however, bear in mind that, in case of a future need for a mastectomy, this type of breast reconstruction will no longer be available.

15

CONTRALATERAL BREAST SURGERY

Contralateral breast surgery aims to correct asymmetry between the operated breast and the contralateral one. Contralateral surgery involves one of the following procedures: (i) adjustment of nipple areola complex; (ii) mastopexy (a procedure that lifts the breast and increases projection); (iii) reduction mammoplasty (breast reduction); or (iv) augmentation mammoplasty (breast enlargement).[9]

IMMEDIATE VERSUS DELAYED

Contralateral oncoplastic surgery can be done either at the same time as breast cancer surgery or as a delayed setting.[10] It may become apparent at the stage of doing the oncoplastic procedure on the side affected with cancer that symmetry cannot be achieved without contralateral reduction. Being aware of this possibility will ensure that the contralateral breast reduction can be done at the same sitting, which would avoid further major surgery and a second general anaesthetic.

Some surgeons prefer doing contralateral surgery as a delayed setting when the final shape of the reconstructed breast is better known. Delayed contralateral surgery is also performed when the volume of the reconstructed breast is difficult to predict, particularly in patients requiring radiotherapy.

For tumours involving the lower medial or lower lateral part of a large ptotic breast, inferior pedicle based breast reduction may be used and symmetry could be achieved by performing a similar procedure on the contralateral breast.[9]

Minor asymetry in the position of nipple-areola complex can be corrected using a circumferential zone of de-epithelisation. Greater degrees of asymmetry requires a mastopexy to achieve symmetry.[9] Slight asymmetry in the position of the nipple–areola complex can be corrected using a crescentric zone of de-epithelisation. Greater degrees of asymmetry of nipple position can be corrected by mastopexy.

The final decision regarding the choice of the oncoplasic procedures employed to achieve symmetry and whether contralateral surgery is performed at the time of undertaking primary surgery (immediate procedure) or as a delayed setting should be made after detailed counselling, taking into consideration patient expectations and objective assessment by the oncoplastic breast surgeon.

CONCLUSIONS

In this era of oncoplastic breast surgery, it would be unreasonable to remove a breast lesion and allow a seroma to fill the wound resulting in subsequent deformity. There is clearly a growing demand for cosmetically acceptable breast conserving surgery the world-over. Breast cancer surgery must be carried out with due consideration to cosmetic outcome without oncological compomise as disfiguring and mutilating excisions are neither justified nor acceptable (Fig. 25).

Oncoplastic breast surgery is an innovative and sophisticated subspecialty within breast surgery and is an essentil skill for the dedicated breast specialist.

We would like to end with a quotation from Prof. Umberto Veronesi, who is considered to be the 'godfather' of modern breast surgery:

Women aware of breast cancer issues and who participate in early detection programmes should be rewarded with gentle and appropriate care and not punished with heavy and often unjustified treatments.

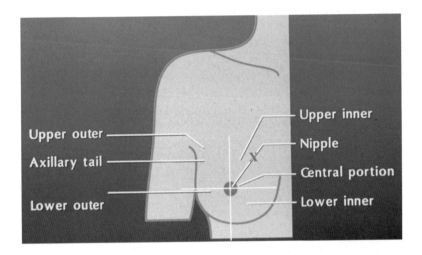

Fig. 1 Round block technique for cancers in the upper inner quadrant of the breast. (Reproduced by permission from Informa Healthcare, *Textbook of Oncoplastic Breast Surgery*, 2004)

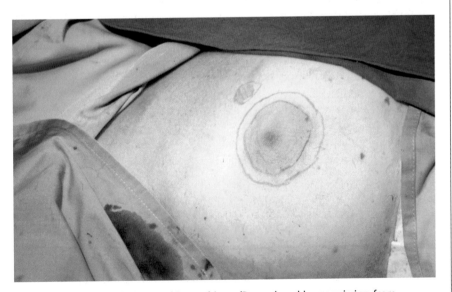

Fig. 2 Round block technique – skin marking. (Reproduced by permission from Informa Healthcare, *Textbook of Oncoplastic Breast Surgery*, 2004)

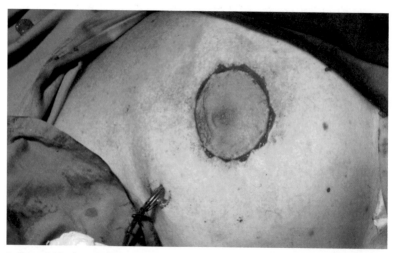

Fig. 3 Round block technique – view after completion of operation. (Reproduced by permission from Informa Healthcare, *Textbook of Oncoplastic Breast Surgery*, 2004)

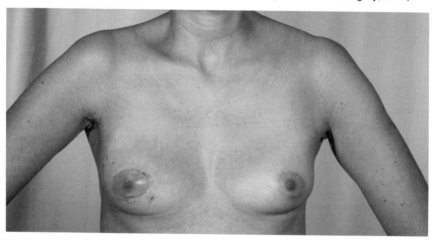

Fig. 4 Round block technique – postoperative view. (Reproduced by permission from Informa Healthcare, *Textbook of Oncoplastic Breast Surgery*, 2004)

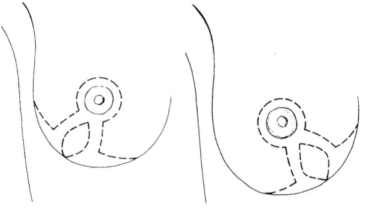

Fig. 5 Comma-shaped breast mammoplasty breast reduction or mastoplexy. (Reproduced by permission from Informa Healthcare, *Textbook of Oncoplastic Breast Surgery*, 2004)

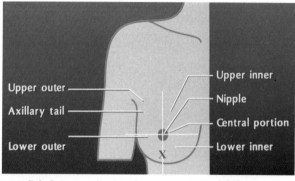

Fig. 6 Superior pedicle breast reduction for cancers in the lower part of the breast. (Reproduced by permission from Informa Healthcare, *Textbook of Oncoplastic Breast Surgery*, 2004)

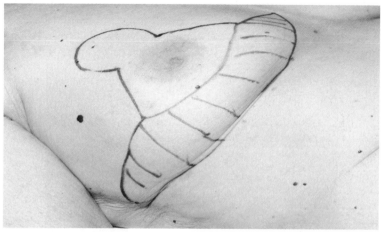

Fig. 7 Superior pedicle breast reduction – skin marking and extent of excision. (Reproduced by permission from Informa Healthcare, *Textbook of Oncoplastic Breast Surgery*, 2004)

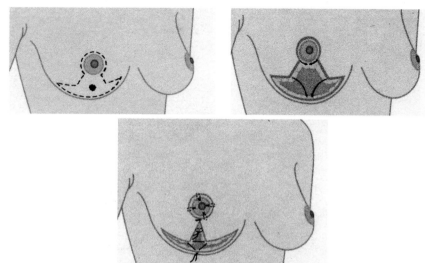

Fig. 8 Superior pedicle breast reduction. (Reproduced by permission from Informa Healthcare, *Textbook of Oncoplastic Breast Surgery*, 2004)

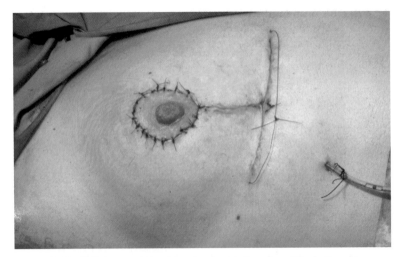

Fig. 9 Superior pedicle breast reduction – postoperative view. (Reproduced by permission from Informa Healthcare, *Textbook of Oncoplastic Breast Surgery*, 2004)

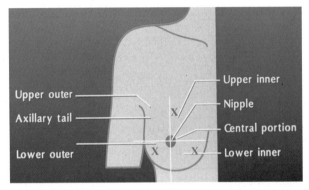

Fig. 10 Inferior pedicle breast reduction for cancers above the nipple or in the lower medial or lateral quadrants. (Reproduced by permission from Informa Healthcare, *Textbook of Oncoplastic Breast Surgery*, 2004)

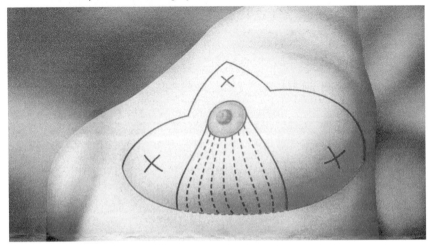

Fig. 11 Inferior pedicle breast reduction. Dotted lines represent the inferior pedicle and 'X' the extent of excision (reduction). (Reproduced by permission from Informa Healthcare, *Textbook of Oncoplastic Breast Surgery*, 2004)

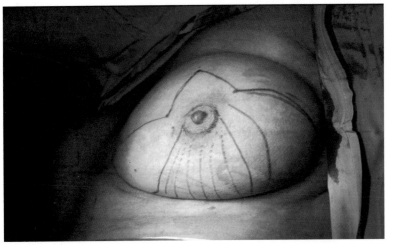

Fig. 12 Inferior pedicle breast reduction – skin marking and extent of excision. (Reproduced by permission from Informa Healthcare, *Textbook of Oncoplastic Breast Surgery*, 2004)

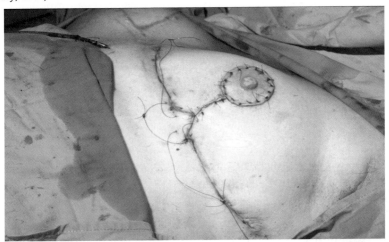

Fig. 13 Inferior pedicle breast reduction – postoperative view. (Reproduced by permission from Informa Healthcare, *Textbook of Oncoplastic Breast Surgery*, 2004)

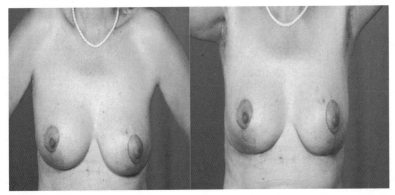

Fig. 14 Inferior pedicle breast reduction – postoperative view with contralateral reduction. (Reproduced by permission from Informa Healthcare, *Textbook of Oncoplastic Breast Surgery*, 2004)

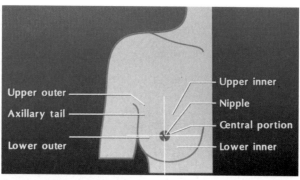

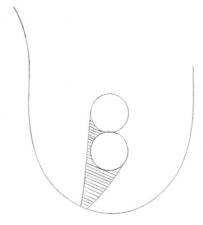

Fig. 15 Grisotti advancement (rotation flap) for central quadrant tumours. (Reproduced by permission from Informa Healthcare, *Textbook of Oncoplastic Breast Surgery*, 2004)

Fig. 16 Grisotti advancement – Line diagram. (Reproduced by permission from Informa Healthcare, *Textbook of Oncoplastic Breast Surgery*, 2004)

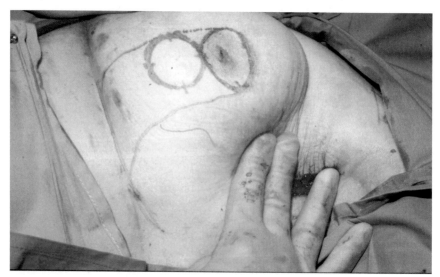

Fig. 17 Grisotti advancement – skin marking. (Reproduced by permission from Informa Healthcare, *Textbook of Oncoplastic Breast Surgery*, 2004)

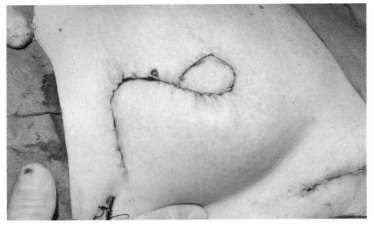

Fig. 18 Grisotti advancement – wound completely closed. (Reproduced by permission from Informa Healthcare, *Textbook of Oncoplastic Breast Surgery*, 2004)

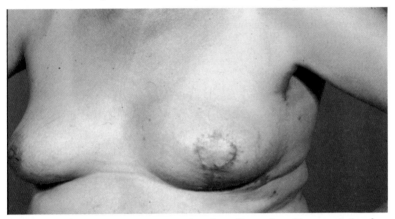

Fig. 19 Grisotti advancement – postoperative view. (Reproduced by permission from Informa Healthcare, *Textbook of Oncoplastic Breast Surgery*, 2004)

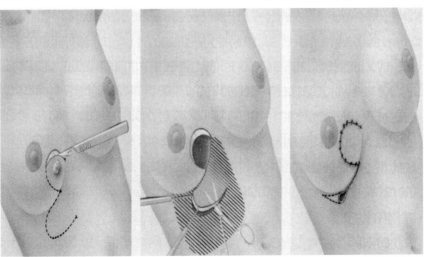

Fig. 20 Thoraco-epigastric flap after breast-conserving surgery. (Reproduced by permission from Informa Healthcare, *Textbook of Oncoplastic Breast Surgery*, 2004)

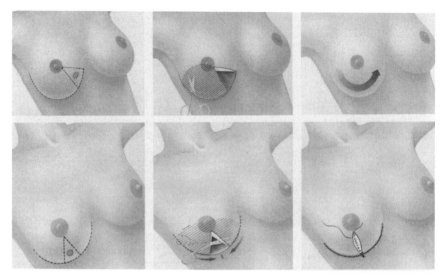

Fig. 21 Glandular rotation after breast-conserving surgery. (Reproduced by permission from Informa Healthcare, *Textbook of Oncoplastic Breast Surgery*, 2004)

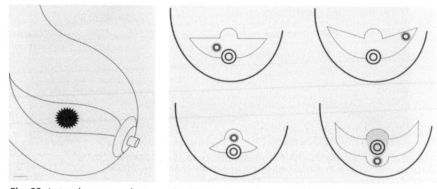

Fig. 22 Lateral mammoplasty.   Fig. 23 Horizontal mammoplasty.
(Reproduced by permission from Informa Healthcare, *Textbook of Oncoplastic Breast Surgery*, 2004)

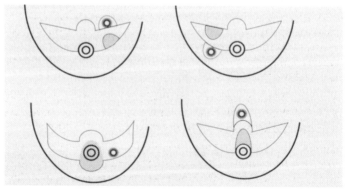

Fig. 24 Horizontal mammoplasty. (Reproduced by permission from Informa Healthcare, *Textbook of Oncoplastic Breast Surgery*, 2004)

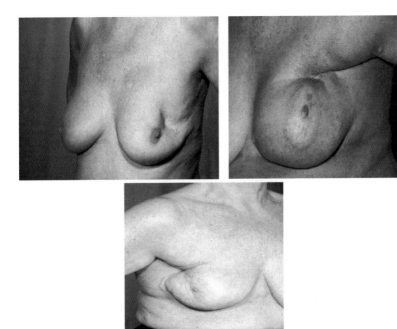

Fig. 25 Poor outcomes following breast-conserving surgery. (Reproduced by permission from Informa Healthcare, *Textbook of Oncoplastic Breast Surgery*, 2004)

Key points for clinical practice

- Over recent years, breast cancer care has been enhanced by the emergence of the specialist breast surgeon with training in oncoplastic surgical skills – the oncoplastic breast surgeon.

- The aims of oncoplastic surgery are wide local excision of the cancer coupled with partial reconstruction of the defect to achieve a cosmetically good result. Avoidance of mastectomy and consequent reduction of psychological morbidity are the principal goals in the development of various oncoplastic techniques.

- Oncoplastic surgery should not be confused with breast reconstructive surgery after mastectomy. The oncoplastic breast surgeon requires the combination of knowledge in thee different specialties: – surgical oncology, plastic surgery and breast radiology.

- Proper patient selection and careful planning after proper radio-logical and clinical assessment are the two essential prerequisites before undertaking oncoplastic breast-conserving surgery.

- Bad cosmetic outcome following breast-conserving surgery occurs due to a combination of factors such as wrongly placed incision, poor surgical technique resulting in local glandular defect and scar contracture.

Key points for clinical practice (continued)

- The primary aim of contralateral breast surgery is to achieve symmetry between the operated breast and the contralateral one, which can be done at the same time as breast cancer surgery or as a delayed setting.

- Extensive resection in the breast could be replaced with volume (volume replacement procedure). The mini latissimus dorsi flap is commonly used to cover these defects. The clinician and the patient must, however, bear in mind that, in case of a future need for a mastectomy, this type of breast reconstruction will no longer be available.

- Good cosmetic outcome can be obtained if deeper glandular tissue is approximated to obliterate glandular defect. After excision of the lesion, the breast tissue must be mobilised at the level of the pectoral fascia and the subcutaneous plane to allow tension-free approximation of tissues.

- Oncoplastic surgery involves both volume displacement and volume replacement techniques. The indications for cosmetically acceptable breast-conserving surgery can be safely extended to tumours involving all the quadrants of the breast, thus expanding the armamentarium of oncoplastic surgery.

- The use of plastic surgical techniques not only ensures good cosmetic outcome, but also allows the cancer surgeon to remove the tumour with greater volume of surrounding tissue, thus extending the boundaries of breast-conserving surgery.

References

1. Skillman JM, Humzah MD, Brown IM et al. The future of breast surgery: a new subspecialty of oncoplastic breast surgeons. Breast 2003; 12: 161–162.
2. Dobson AR. Subspecialty of oncoplastic breast surgery is needed to meet demand. BMJ 2003; 326: 1165–1167.
3. McGlothin TDQ. Breast surgery as a specialized practice. Am J Surg 2005; 190: 264–268.
4. Fisher B, Anderson S, Bryant J et al. Twenty year follow up of a randomized trial comparing total mastectomy, lumpectomy and lumpectomy plus radiation for treatment of invasive breast cancer. N Engl J Med 2002; 347: 1233–1241.
5. Veronesi U, Cascinelli N, Mariani L et al. Twenty year follow up of randomized study comparing breast conserving surgery with radical mastectomy for early breast cancer. N Engl J Med 2002; 347: 1227–1232.
6. Clarke M, Collins R, Darby S et al. Effects of radiotherapy and extent of surgery for early breast cancer on local recurrence and 15 year survival: an overview of randomized trials. Lancet 2005; 366: 2087–2106.
7. Petit J, Youssef O, Garusi C. (eds) Oncoplastic and Reconstructive Surgery of the Breast, Vol. 10. New York: Taylor Francis, 2004; 101.
8. Petit J, Youssef O, Garusi C. (eds) Oncoplastic and Reconstructive Surgery of the Breast, Vol. 10. New York: Taylor Francis, 2004; 102–109.
9. Nannelli A, Calabrese C, Cataliotti L, Querci della Rovere G. (eds) Oncoplastic and Reconstructive Surgery of the Breast, Vol. 12. New York: Taylor Francis, 2004; 115–125.
10. Masetti R, Pirulli PG, Magno S et al. Oncoplastic techniques in conservative surgical treatment of the breast. Breast Cancer 2000; 7: 276–280.

Bubby Thava Robert B. Galland

3

Novel therapies for varicose veins

Varicose veins have a significant impact on Western society, affecting 32% of women and 40% of men.[1] Common symptoms include aching, heaviness, ankle swelling, pruritis and, sometimes, muscle cramps. These symptoms are often made worse by prolonged standing or warm weather. Increased referrals for varicose vein treatment have been noted in summer months.[2] Long-standing chronic venous insufficiency can result in skin changes which include eczema, pigmentation, lipodermatosclerosis and ulceration. Cosmetic concerns relate to the varicose veins themselves and any associated skin changes.

Surgical treatment of varicose veins has been the gold standard for many years. Over the last few years, alternatives to surgery have been introduced which have caught the public imagination. Paradoxically, during the time that these techniques have been introduced, primary care trusts in the UK have started to ration varicose vein treatment such that significantly fewer patients are now being offered treatment than a few years ago. In our unit, this has resulted in a reduction in varicose vein procedures of about 80%.[3]

The principles and results of conventional operation and novel techniques are discussed.

SURGICAL TREATMENT

PRINCIPLE

Proximal ligation and stripping deal with superficial reflux and avulsions remove non-truncal varicose veins.

Bubby Thava MA MRCS
Specialist Registrar, Department of Vascular Surgery, Royal Berkshire Hospital, Reading RG1 5AN, UK

Robert B. Galland MD FRCS (for correspondence)
Consultant Surgeon, Department of Vascular Surgery, Royal Berkshire Hospital, Reading RG1 5AN, UK.
E-mail: robert.galland@royalberkshire.nhs.uk

KEY POINTS OF TECHNIQUE

The procedure is usually done under general anaesthetic as a day case. The saphenofemoral junction (SFJ) is in a fairly constant position lying in the groin crease immediately medial to the femoral artery pulse. The saphenopopliteal junction (SPJ), on the other hand, is in a variable position in the popliteal fossa at a variable depth from the skin surface. Marking the uppermost palpable short saphenous trunk and duplex marking of the SPJ allows accurate pre-operative planning. The junction usually lies in the upper outer part of the popliteal fossa.[4,5] Stripping the long saphenous vein (LSV) reduces the risk of postoperative recurrence.[6] Perforation invagination (PIN) stripping is preferred to the more traumatic conventional stripping using an 'acorn'. Concerns that short saphenous stripping is associated with an increased risk of nerve damage are probably unfounded. Stab avulsions are used to remove remaining varicose veins which should have been carefully marked pre-operatively.

RESULTS

Varicose vein operations have been shown to improve quality of life significantly.[7,8] Up to 50% recurrence rate at 10 years has been reported.[6] However, many patients are not aware or not concerned about those recurrences and remain pleased with the results.

COMPLICATIONS

- As with any surgical procedure involving an anaesthetic there is a mortality associated with the varicose vein operations. This is of the order of 1 per 10,000.

- Bruising, especially in the lower medial thigh following stripping, can be extensive and painful. Nevertheless, recovery is generally quick with most patients being back to normal within 2 weeks.[9]

- Wound infection and lymph leaks have been reported in 2.8% and 0.5%, respectively.[10]

- Thrombo-embolism is uncommon but can be fatal. Clinical evidence of deep vein thrombosis (DVT) is reported in 0.15–0.5% of cases.[10,11] However, the incidence is found to be much higher if scanning is carried out postoperatively, this being approximately 5%. Most of these DVTs remain asymptomatic.[12]

- The commonest cause of litigation following varicose vein procedures is nerve damage.[13] Stripping of the long saphenous vein can produce numbness around the medial malleolus. This may be reduced by stripping to knee rather than ankle. Wood et al.[14] identified numbness or paraesthesia in 17 (27%) limbs at 6-week follow-up. It was found that 11 (17%) limbs were affected below the knee and 7 (11%) limbs were affected at the thigh or groin.[14]

- Avulsions are also associated with nerve injury. The common peroneal nerve as it passes around the neck of the fibula is particularly vulnerable.

POWERED PHLEBECTOMY

PRINCIPLE

The procedure is carried out under general anaesthetic. Illumination of varices is carried out by inserting a light source into subcutaneous fat through a 1-cm incision. A phlebectomy device is inserted through another incision which removes veins over a 5 cm area using a rotating blade which also provides suction.[15] It was hoped that reduced bruising and risk of infection with a better cosmetic result could be achieved by a smaller number of 1-cm incisions rather than many 2–3 mm hook phlebectomy incisions. The TriVex system (Smith and Nephew Inc.; Andover, MA, USA) is the device most commonly used.

RESULTS

One randomised, controlled trial has shown no advantage for powered phlebectomy over conventional surgery with regard to cosmesis. It has an advantage of a reduced operative time in extensive varicosities with significantly fewer incisions.[16]

Any small advantage in the procedure being quicker compared with conventional phlebectomies is more than offset by the increased costs of the procedure. The disposables used for TriVex can cost up to 262 euros.

> ## Key point 1
> • Operation is a gold standard but morbidity is encountered particularly with regard to the groin incision and stripping. Re-operation involving the saphenofemoral junction or saphenopopliteal junction can be difficult.

NOVEL TECHNIQUES

Novel techniques have been found to be as good as surgery in producing LSV occlusion in the short term. Javid et al.[17] compared radiofrequency/laser ablation and cryosurgery against high tie and ligation. It was suggested that these novel techniques may confer a benefit in postoperative pain and oedema.[17]

RADIOFREQUENCY ABLATION (RFA)

PRINCIPLE

The aim is to obliterate the LSV, thereby stopping reflux without the necessity of a groin incision and proximal ligation. Duplex scanning has shown that if veins are less than 5 mm from the underside of the dermis, tumescent anaesthesia using a solution of saline and lignocaine can protect surrounding structures. Up to 250 ml of a 0.2% solution of lignocaine neutralised with sodium bicarbonate can be used.[18] Avulsions would still need to be carried out. Thermal injury to the LSV results in collagen denaturation without destroying vessel wall integrity. Obliteration leaves behind a small thrombus plug which effectively isolates the closed segment.[19] The vein wall temperature is monitored and held at a constant 85°C by a feedback mechanism. The most commonly used closure system is VNUS Closure (VNUS Medical Technologies; San Jose, CA, USA).

KEY POINTS OF TECHNIQUE

A guidewire is inserted into the LSV at knee level. A 6-F or 8-F sheath plus VNUS catheter is passed to the SFJ under duplex guidance. A tourniquet is then applied. Bipolar electrodes at the end of the venous catheter allow controlled heating of the LSV so leading to damage of the vein wall and closure of the lumen. The catheter is then pulled back in a controlled fashion.

The majority of patients require additional therapy. In a study by Almeida et al.,[26] avulsions were carried out in 88% and sclerotherapy in 16% of limbs treated.

RESULTS

Early treatment failure could be associated with fast catheter pull-back rates. This brief exposure to thermal injury can achieve endothelial destruction with incomplete wall contraction which results in thrombosis but not necessarily obliteration.[20] Immediate LSV occlusion is achieved in 85–100% of cases (Table

Table 1 Typical results of radiofrequency ablation as adapted from Almeida et al. (2006)[31]

Reference	Limbs (n)	Skin burn (%)	Paraes- thesia (%)	Phleb- itis (%)	DVT (%)	PE (%)	In. Ob. rates	Recanal- isation (%)	Mean follow- up
Weiss et al. (2002)[21]	140	0	4	0	0	0	98	10	9 mths
Merchant et al. (2002)[22]	318	4	15	2	1	1	93	15	24 mths
Rautio et al. (2002)[23]	30	3	10	6	0	0	100	17	10 mths
Lurie et al. (2003)[24]	44	2	23	4	0	0	95	10	4 mths
Hingorini et al. (2004)[25]	73	0	0	0.3	16	0	96	4	10 days
Almeida et al. (2004)[26]	106	0	2	NA	0	0	85	8	3 mths
Nicolini et al. (2004)[27]	330	N/A	2.5–7.5	0	0	0	N/A	12%	3 yrs
Merchant et al. (2005)[28]	1078	2	12	3	0.5	1		11	4 yrs
Hinchliffe et al. (2005)[29]	16	0	19	6	0	0		13	1 yr
Perala et al. (2005)[30]	15	0	7	7	0	0	93	0	3 yrs
Almeida et al. (2006)[31]	128	2	N/A	0	N/A	0	85	5	3 yrs

In. Ob. rates = Initial obliteration rates; mths = months; yrs = years.

1) Recanalisation occurs with time and may, or may not, be associated with recurrent varicose veins. LSV recanalisation has been reported in 15% of cases within 1 year of complete occlusion.[26] Most of these recanalisations occurred within a year. These results were inferior to laser treatment. A 12% recanalisation rate was seen by Nicolini et al.[27] at 3 years. Recurrent varicose veins at 1- and 2-year follow-up have been reported in 14% of cases.[24]

In a small, randomised, controlled trial involving patients with recurrent varicose veins, operation time, pain and bruising were all lower in VNUS compared with revision groin surgery and stripping.[29]

COMPLICATIONS

- Paraesthesae are reported in up to 20% of cases. When comparisons have been made, this is generally higher than that seen in patients undergoing operation. The risk of paraesthesae appears to be higher if the LSV is ablated to the ankle rather than the knee.[28] The rate of skin burns is very variable ranging between zero and approximately 20%. There is little information on the long-term consequences of this complication. As described earlier, if the vein is close to the dermis tumescent anaesthesia may reduce the risk of burns.

- DVT has been reported in up to 16% of cases with the occasional pulmonary embolus being described. The higher association with venous thrombosis compared with operative methods may be because of propagation of the LSV thrombus into the common femoral vein. In one study, prospective duplex scanning showed a tongue of thrombus extending into the common femoral vein in 11 of 66 patients.[25]

RESULTS COMPARED WITH OTHER MODALITIES

A study comparing EVLT with RFA showed a significantly higher efficacy in favour of EVLT when looking at recanalisation rates (2.3% versus 7.5%). However, RFA is associated with lower levels of postoperative thrombophlebitis. Historically, RFA has been associated with higher rates of skin burns and paraesthesia which have largely been eliminated with the advent of tumescent analgesia.[31]

ADVANTAGES OVER OPERATION

Compared with operation, RFA results in less pain and quicker return to normal activities.[23,24] Perala et al.[30] showed an increase in rate of recanalisation from 1.7% at 1 week to 11.3% at 2 years. It may be of value in recurrent varicose veins avoiding a potential difficult groin dissection.

Key point 2
- Radiofrequency ablation is more rapid and associated with less morbidity than operation as groin dissection is avoided. It can also be completed under local anaesthetic and so there is a much quicker return to normal activities.

ENDOVENOUS LASER THERAPY (EVLT)

PRINCIPLE

This can be carried out under local or general anaesthesia. EVLT involves delivery of laser energy directly into the blood vessel lumen. Non-thrombotic vein occlusion is achieved by heating the vein wall. Different wavelengths, different energies and pulsed or continuous light have been used. There is no feedback control as with RFA, so energy is delivered at a predetermined rate. With sufficient heating of the vein wall there is endothelial denudation and collagen contraction. This results in the vein thrombosing.[32]

KEY POINTS OF TECHNIQUE

Using duplex ultrasound, the SFJ and LSV in the thigh are marked pre-operatively. One method involves aseptic perigenicular cannulation of the LSV with the patient in the reverse Trendelenburg position. A catheter is then introduced (5-F) to align the tip at the SFJ. The patient then has a sterile bare tipped 600 μm laser fibre introduced via this catheter for laser ablation of the LSV.

RESULTS

Immediate occlusion is achieved in 90% of cases (Table 2). Data on long-term canalisation rates are limited but Min et al.[32] described a 2% recanalisation rate at 6 months. Darwood et al.[1] showed a rate of 2% at 1 year. Rasmussen et al.[18] showed a recanalisation rate of 4% at 6 months.

COMPLICATIONS

- The incidence of skin burns and paraesthesia vary depending upon wavelength used and whether tumescent anaesthesia is used. Proebstle et al.[35] reported bruising and induration in all of 36 limbs treated and resultant hyperpigmentation in 3%. Others have noted in a series of 244 legs that skin burns were present in 4.8% and paraesthesae in 36.5%.[36]

Table 2 Typical results of endovenous laser therapy adapted from Almeida et al. (2006)[31]

Reference	Limbs (n)	Skin burn (%)	Paraes-thesia (%)	Phleb-itis (%)	DVT (%)	PE (%)	In. Ob. rates (%)	Recanal-isation (%)	Mean follow-up
Min et al. (2003)[32]	504	0	0	5	0	0	98	2	6 mths
Pugioni et al. (2005)[33]	77	N/A	N/A	4	2	0	94	4	1 mths
Almeida et al. (2006)[31]	819	N/A	0.2	N/A	0.2	N/A	92	2	6 mths
Rasmussen et al. (2007)[18]	121	N/A	1	2	1	0		4	6 mths
Darwood et al. (2008)[1]	42	0	0	14	0	0	98	2	1 yr

In. Ob. rates = Initial obliteration rates; mths = months; yr = year.

- The rate of clinically detected DVT following the EVLT is low (0–1%).[26,31] In a review of series and RCTs, there was only one report of a pulmonary embolus.[28] However, in a study of 39 patients undergoing early post-operative duplex scanning, three were found to have thrombus extending into the common femoral vein.[33]

- Gibson et al.[37] demonstrated EVLT to be an effective technique for eliminating short saphenous vein (SSV) reflux. The study showed that 96% of short saphenous trunks stayed closed at 17 months and only 1.6% had paraesthesia at the lateral malleolus at 6 weeks follow up.[37]

- The incidence of DVTs was found to be higher than in surgical series with DVT noted in 12 limbs (5.7%) at 1-week follow-up. It was postulated by the authors that the configuration of the SPJ was the only factor predictive of DVTs in these cases.

Key point 3

- Endovenous laser therapy has similar outcomes to surgery and can also be performed under local anaesthetic. However, it is more

---

FOAM SCLEROTHERAPY

PRINCIPLE

Duplex-guided foam sclerotherapy is a variation of liquid sclerotherapy. The liquid sclerosant is mixed with air, carbon dioxide or oxygen to create the foam. It is then injected into the LSV. The advantage of foam over liquid is that it allows a smaller quantity of sclerosant to cover a greater surface area so pushing blood from the vein.[38]

KEY POINTS OF TECHNIQUE

The Tessari method is the most commonly used. Two syringes are connected by a three-way tap. Fluid sclerosant is forcibly mixed with air and froth to produce a foam. The most commonly used agent is polidocanol (3% with varying volumes, depending on vessel diameter, of 2–2.5 ml). Sodium tetradecyl sulphate can also be used. Strength of agent and volume used depends on vessel diameter. A needle is inserted into the long saphenous vein at the level of the knee perforator and, under duplex guidance, foam is injected to fill the entire long saphenous vein. The top of the LSV is then compressed to keep foam contained within the LSV. Foam can be visualised with duplex scanning which confers better results for GSV occlusion.[39]

RESULTS

Initial technical success in obliterating the LSV is achieved in 88–97% of studies. Jia et al.,[39] in a review involving 69 studies of foam sclerotherapy, found that long-term venous occlusion was maintained in about 85% of cases (range, 67–94%). However, the follow-up for most of these studies was less than 3 years. Recurrence of varicose veins was about 8% (range, 1–15%). The duration of studies providing these data was 6 weeks to 6 years. It has been estimated that the recurrence rate is 50% at 10 years.

COMPLICATIONS

- The risk of DVT and pulmonary embolus is less than 1% (range, 0–6%).[39]

- Thrombophlebitis occurs in about 5% and skin necrosis in 1.3%.[39] Of concern is the pigmentation which affects nearly 20% of limbs undergoing foam sclerotherapy. This pigmentation may take months to improve and may never go completely.

- However, the main concern following foam sclerotherapy is foam micro-embolism, which is reported to occur 'commonly'.[40] In the presence of a patent foramen ovale, which is present in 10% of the population, this can potentially lead to neurological symptoms. If there is a patent foramen ovale, microemboli in the middle cerebral artery have been seen in 90% of patients.[41] Visual disturbances (possibly as a result of microemboli or foam-induced migraine) have been reported in 0–6% of series. None of these symptoms have lasted more than 2 h. However, several strokes and transient ischaemic attacks have now been reported.[42,43] In view of this, the UK National Institute for Health and Clinical Excellence (NICE) is currently (November 2008) reviewing evidence on foam sclerotherapy and may amend the original report which was published in May 2007.[39] Should neurological events occur following foam sclerotherapy it has been suggested that an echocardiogram should be carried out to search for a patent foramen ovale. This should, perhaps, be routine procedure before any patient undergoes foam sclerotherapy.

- An alternative to foam sclerotherapy of the long saphenous trunk alone might be to combine it with saphenofemoral ligation under local anaesthetic.[44] The foam could be delivered under ultrasound guidance from knee level; alternatively, an umbilical catheter could be inserted down the long saphenous vein at the time of the SFL. The risk of foam micro-embolism should at least be reduced with this technique.

- Anaphylaxis has also been reported following foam sclerotherapy.

RESULTS COMPARED WITH OTHER MODALITIES

When compared with operation, liquid sclerotherapy was effective for varicosities secondary to incompetent perforators below the knees. However, operation was more effective in the presence of saphenofemoral or saphenopopliteal incompetence.[45] Yamaki et al.[47] achieved complete LSV occlusion in 67.6% of cases with foam compared with 17.5% with liquid.

ADVANTAGES

The major advantage of foam sclerotherapy is that is can be carried out under local anaesthetic as an 'office' procedure. It can also be easily repeated.

> ### Key point 4
> - Foam sclerotherapy is cost effective and can be performed under local anaesthetic in the 'office' setting. However, it can be associated with serious adverse effects such as strokes and visual disturbances.

CRYOSURGERY

PRINCIPLE

The point of this technique is to avoid a distal incision to remove the stripper. A cryoprobe placed within the vein is cooled with NO_2 or CO_2 to a temperature of –85°C. The vein freezes to the probe and can be retrogradely stripped after 5 s of freezing.

KEY POINTS IN TECHNIQUE

A probe is passed down the long saphenous vein following saphenofemoral ligation.

RESULTS

Providing that the vein is stripped out, these should be no different to conventional proximal ligation and stripping.

COMPLICATIONS

- There seem to be no specific complications as a result of the cryosurgery technique.

ADVANTAGES

There is a reduced operating time compared with conventional stripping.[48] It is also thought to be advantageous in obese patients as the technique is easier than conventional stripping. Its main disadvantage is cost, which makes its general usage largely prohibitive.

RESULTS COMPARED WITH OTHER MODALITIES

Pain scores have been found to be significantly higher in the short term for cryosurgery compared to traditional stripping[48] and EVLT.[49] Patients are able to resume normal activities within 8 days,[48] which is significantly less than EVLT.[49]

Documented severe outcomes are rare. Wound infection or thrombo-phlebitis are the most commonly associated complications. Longer term studies show that EVLT and cryostripping are similarly effective. Quality-of-life measures show a distinct disadvantage to cryostripping.[28]

Key point 5

- Cryostripping is an easier technique than conventional stripping so conferring an advantage in elderly or overweight patients. It is, however, more expensive than surgery.

Key points for clinical practice

- Operation is a gold standard but morbidity is encountered parti-cularly with regard to the groin incision and stripping. Re-operation involving the saphenofemoral junction or saphenopopliteal junction can be difficult.

- Radiofrequency ablation is more rapid and associated with less morbidity than operation as groin dissection is avoided. It can also be completed under local anaesthetic and so there is a much quicker return to normal activities.

- Endovenous laser therapy has similar outcomes to surgery and can also be performed under local anaesthetic. However, it is more expensive and there is a higher risk of deep vein thromboses.

- Foam sclerotherapy is cost effective and can be performed under local anaesthetic in the 'office' setting. However, it can be associated with serious adverse effects such as strokes and visual disturbances.

- Cryostripping is an easier technique than conventional stripping so conferring an advantage in elderly or overweight patients. It is, however, more expensive than surgery.

Acknowledgement

Presented at the Association of Surgeons meeting, Bournemouth, May 2008

References

1. Darwood RJ, Theivacumar N, Dellagrammaticas D, Mavor D, Gough MJ. Randomised clinical trial comparing endovenous laser ablation with surgery for the treatment of primary great saphenous varicose veins. *Br J Surg* 2008; **95**: 294–301.
2. Cook TA, Michaels JA, Galland RB. Varicose vein clinics: modelling the effects of seasonal variation in referrals. *J R Coll Surg Edinb* 1997; **42**: 400–402.
3. Bajwa A, Magee TR, Galland RB. Reduction in varicose vein services: impact on operative training. *Ann R Coll Surg Engl* 2007; **89**: 789–791.
4. Aiono S, Simmons MJ, Magee TR, Galland RB. The significance of a palpable short saphenous vein in the popliteal fossa: a useful clinical sign. *Phlebology* 1999; **14**: 84.

5. Pittathankal AA, Richards T, Magee TR, Galland RB. If the short saphenous vein is palpable in the popliteal fossa is a duplex scan required for the accurate pre-operative localisation of the sapheno-popliteal junction? *Phlebology* 2002; **17**: 78.

6. Winterborn RJ, Foy C, Earnshaw JJ. Causes of varicose vein recurrence: late results of a randomized controlled trial of stripping the long saphenous vein. *J Vasc Surg* 2004; **40**: 634–639.

7. MacKenzie RK, Paisley A, Allan PL *et al.* The effect of long saphenous vein stripping on the quality of life – a randomised trial. *J Vasc Surg* 2002; **35**: 1197–1203.

8. Durkin MT, Turton EPL, Wijesinghe LD *et al.* Long saphenous vein stripping and quality of life – a randomised trial. *Eur J Vasc Surg* 2001; **21**: 545–549.

9. Bailey CMH, Perkins JMT, Garnett S *et al.* Evidence-based follow-up after varicose veins surgery. *Phlebology* 2002; **16**: 170–172.

10. Critchley G, Handa A, Maw A, Harvey A, Harvey MR, Corbett CRR. Complications of varicose vein surgery. *Ann R Coll Surg Engl* 1997; **79**: 105–110.

11. Keith Jr LN, Smead WL. Saphenous vein stripping and its complications. *Surg Clin North Am* 1983; **63**: 1303–1312.

12. Van Rij AM, Hill GB, Christie RA. Incidence of deep vein thrombosis after varicose vein surgery. *Br J Surg* 2004; **91**: 1582–1585.

13. Campbell WB, France F, Goodwin HM. Medicolegal claims in vascular surgery. *Ann R Coll Surg Engl* 2002; **84**: 181–184.

14. Wood JJ, Chant H, Lugharne M, Chant T, Mitchell C. A prospective study of cutaneous nerve injury following long saphenous vein injury. *Eur J Vasc Endovasc Surg* 2005; **30**: 654–658.

15. Arumugasamy M, McGreal G, O'Connor FL. The technique of transluminated powered phlebectomy (TPP) – novel, minimally invasive system for varicose vein surgery. *Eur J Vasc Endovasc Surg* 2002; **23**: 180–182.

16. Aremu MA, Mahendran B, Butcher W *et al.* A prospective randomised trial: conventional versus powered phlebectomy. *J Vasc Surg* 2004; **39**: 88–94.

17. Javid M, Lovegrove R, Magee T, Galland RB. Treatment of long saphenous varicose veins: a meta-analysis of novel therapies versus conventional surgery.

18. Rasmussen LH, Bjoern L, Lawaetz M *et al.* Randomised trial comparing endovenous laser ablation of the great saphenous vein with high ligation and stripping in patients with varicose veins: Short term results. *J Vasc Surg* 2007; **46**: 308–314.

19. McDaniel MD, Nehler MR, Santilli SM *et al.* Extended outcome assessment in the care of vascular diseases: revising the paradigm for the 21st century. *J Vasc Surg* 2000; **32**: 1239–1250.

20. Manfrini S, Gasbarro V, Danielson G *et al.* Endovenous management of saphenous vein reflux. *J Vasc Surg* 2000; **32**: 330–341.

21. Weiss RA, Wiess MA. Controlled radiofrequency endovenous occlusion using a unique radio frequency catheter under duplex guidance to eliminate saphenous varicose vein reflux: a two year follow up. *Dermatol Surg* 2002; **28**: 38–42.

22. Merchant RF, DePalma RG, Kabnick LS. Endovascular obliteration of saphenous reflux: a multicenter study. *J Vasc Surg* 2002; **35**: 1190–1196.

23. Rautio T, Ohinmaa A, Perala J *et al.* Endovenous obliteration versus conventional stripping operation in the treatment of primary varicose veins: a randomised controlled trial with comparison of the costs. *J Vasc Surg* 2002; **35**: 958–965.

24. Lurie F, Creton D, Eklof B *et al.* Prospective randomised study of endovenous radiofrequency obliteration (closure) versus ligation and vein stripping (EVOLVeS): two-year follow up. *Eur J Vasc Endovasc Surg* 2005; **29**: 67–73.

25. Hingorani A, Ascher E, Markevisch N *et al.* Deep venous thrombosis after radio frequency ablation of greater saphenous vein: a word of caution. *J Vasc Surg* 2004; **40**: 500–504.

26. Almeida JI. Radiofrequency ablation versus laser ablation in the treatment of varicose veins: value and limitation. *Vascular* 2004; **12**: s57.

27. Nicolini P and The Closure Group. Treatment of primary varicose veins by endovenous obliteration with the venous closure system: results of a prospective multicentre study. *Eur J Vasc Endovasc Surg* 2005; **29**: 433–439.

28. Merchant RF, Pichot O, Myers KA. Four year follow up on endovascular radiofrequency

obliteration of great saphenous reflux. *Dermatol Surg* 2005; **31**: 129–134.

29. Hinchliffe RJ, Ubhi J, Beech A *et al.* A prospective randomised controlled trial of VNUS closure versus surgery for the treatment of recurrent long saphenous varicose veins. *Eur J Vasc Endovasc Surg* 2006; **31**: 212–218.

30. Perala J, Rautio T, Biancari F *et al.* Radiofrequency endovenous obliteration versus stripping of the long saphenous vein in the management of primary varicose veins: 3-year outcome of a randomised study. *Ann Vasc Surg* 2005; **19**: 669–672.

31. Almeida JI, Raines JK. Radiofrequency ablation and laser ablation in the treatment of varicose veins. *Ann Vasc Surg* 2006; **20**: 547–552.

32. Min R, Khilnani N, Zimmet SE. Endovenous laser treatment of saphenous vein reflux: long term results. *J Vasc Interv Radiol* 2003; **14**: 991–996.

33. Puggioni A, Kalra M, Carmo M *et al.* Endovenous laser therapy and radiofrequency ablation of the great saphenous vein: analysis of early efficacy and complications. *J Vasc Surg* 2005; **42**: 488–493.

34. Rasmussen LH, Bjoern L, Lawaetz M *et al.* Randomised trial comparing endovenous laser ablation of the great saphenous vein with high ligation and stripping in patients with varicose veins: Short term results. *J Vasc Surg* 2007; **46**: 308–314.

35. Proebstle M, Guldlehr HA, Kargl A, Knop J. Infrequent early recanalisation of greater saphenous vein after endovenous laser treatment. *J Vasc Surg* 2003; **38**: 511–516.

36. Chang CJ, Chua JJ. Endovenous laser photocoagulation (EVLP) for varicose veins. *Lasers Surg Med* 2002; **31**: 257–262.

37. Gibson KD, Ferris BL, Polissar N, Neradilek B, Pepper D. Endovenous laser treatment of the small saphenous vein: efficacy and complications. *J Vasc Surg* 2007; **45**: 795–801.

38. Beale RJ, Gough MJ. Treatment options for primary varicose veins – a review. *Eur J Vasc Endovasc Surg* 2005; **30**: 36–40.

39. Jia X, Mowatt G, Burr JM, Cassar K, Cook J, Frazer C. Systematic review of foam sclerotherapy for varicose veins. *Br J Surg* 2007; **94**: 925–936.

40. Cuelen RPM, Vernooy K. Reply to letter regarding article titled 'Microembolism during foam sclerotherapy of varicose veins' in the *New England Journal of Medicine*. *Phlebology* 2008; **23**: 23–50.

41. Regan JD, Gibson KD, Ferris B *et al.* Safety of proprietary sclerosant microfoam for saphenous incompetence in patients with R-to-L shunt; interim report. *J Vasc Interv Radiol* 2008; **19 (Suppl)**: 35.

42. Forlee MV, Grouden M, Moore DJ, Shanik G. Stroke after varicose vein foam injection sclerotherapy. *J Vasc Surg* 2006; **43**: 162–164.

43. Bush RG, Derrick M, Manjoney D. Major neurological events following foam sclerotherapy. *Phlebology* 2008; **23**: 189–192.

44. Bountouroglou DG, Azzam M, Kakkos SK, Pathmarajah M, Young P, Geroulakos G. Ultrasound-guided foam sclerotherapy combined with sapheno-femoral ligation compared to surgical treatment of varicose veins: early results of a randomised controlled trial. *Eur J Vasc Endovasc Surg* 2006; **31**: 93–100.

45. Hobbs JT. Surgery and sclerotherapy in the treatment of varicose veins. *Arch Surg* 1974; **109**: 793–796.

46. Rutgers PH, Kitslaa R, Pjeh M. Randomised trial of stripping versus high ligation in the treatment of the incompetent greater saphenous vein. *Am J Surg* 1994; **168**: 311–315.

47. Yamaki T, Motohiro N, Susumu I. Comparative study of duplex-guided foam sclerotherapy and duplex-guided liquid sclerotherapy for the treatment of superficial venous insufficiency. *Dermatol Surg* 2004; **30**: 718–722.

48. Shouten R, Mollen RM, Kuijpers HC. A comparison between cryosurgery and conventional stripping in varicose vein surgery: perioperative features and complications. *Ann Vasc Surg* 2006; **20**: 306–311.

49. Disselhoff BC, der Kinderen DJ, Kelder JC, Moll FL. Randomized clinical trial comparing endovenous laser with cryostripping for great saphenous varicose veins. *Br J Surg* 2008; **95**: 1.

Sanjeev Misra Arun Chaturvedi

4

Management of adult extremity soft tissue sarcomas

Soft tissue sarcomas are an uncommon, heterogeneous group of tumours that account for less than 1% of all adult cancers.[1] Despite their relative rarity, soft tissue sarcomas have interested surgeons, pathologists, radiotherapists and medical oncologists because of their diversity and therapeutic challenge. Three decades ago, management of extremity sarcomas consisted largely of amputations. This practice often resulted in significant patient disability and poor function. Optimum treatment strategies with the goal of limb preservation have evolved substantially over the last two decades.[2] Paediatric soft tissue sarcomas differ from adult soft tissue sarcomas in the approaches to staging and treatment. The present discussion is restricted to adult soft tissue sarcomas occurring in extremities.

Soft tissue sarcomas can occur anywhere in the body but the majority occur in extremities (40% lower extremity and 20% upper extremity). Other less common sites are trunk (10%), retroperitoneal/intraperitoneal (20%), and head and neck (10%).[3]

Key point 1

- Soft tissue sarcomas are a diverse group of malignant tumours with different biological behaviours.

Sanjeev Misra MS MCh FRCS FICS MAMS (for correspondence)
Professor, Department of Surgical Oncology, King George's Medical University, Lucknow, India.
E-mail: misralko@satyam.net.in, misralko@gmail.com

Arun Chaturvedi MS MAMS
Professor and Head, Department of Surgical Oncology, King George's Medical University, Lucknow, India

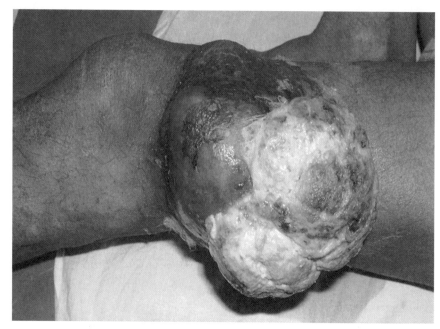

Fig. 1 Fungating soft tissue sarcoma of the thigh.

DIAGNOSIS

CLINICAL PRESENTATION

Soft tissue sarcomas occur in all age groups but are commonest in the fifth and sixth decades of life. Both sexes are equally affected.[4]

The most common presenting symptom in soft tissue sarcomas is of a painless, gradually increasing mass. This may have been present for a variable period of time, usually, less than a year. The size of tumour at diagnosis varies according to the site. Tumours of the distal extremity are usually small as they are likely to be noticed earlier, whereas tumours in the thigh become quite large before they are detected. Size is one of the most important clinical features of a soft tissue lesion. Any soft tissue lesion over 5 cm in maximum diameter has a 20% likelihood of being malignant. Lesions located in the thigh and buttock are more likely to be malignant than in other locations. A deep mass greater than 5 cm in diameter located proximally in the limb in a patient older than 50 years, has a 50% chance of being malignant.[5] The majority of soft tissue sarcomas are painless, but some soft tissue sarcomas such as nerve tumours can be painful or develop pain due to direct invasion or mass effect on adjacent structures. The lack of pain has been identified as one of the reasons for delayed presentation of soft tissue sarcomas. A review from Ireland found a median delay, from initial symptoms to diagnosis, of 28 weeks. The delay was equally attributed to the patient and doctor.[6]

A history of recent trauma is often present. However, the trauma is thought to draw attention to a pre-existing condition, rather than to have a causal association. Patients may also present with pressure symptoms such as distal oedema, motor paralysis and parasthesia. Rarely, the lesion may have broken through the skin when diagnosed (Fig. 1). Systemic symptoms such as fever and weight loss are uncommon. The rate of growth of soft tissue sarcomas varies with the aggressiveness of the tumour. Low-grade tumours may progress over a long period and may be mistaken for benign tumours, especially lipomas.

Physical examination should include the locoregional area and systemic assessment. It is important to determine if the lump is superficial or deep to the fascia as this is essential for management and prognostication. The neurovascular status of the limb should be examined and documented. Nodal metastasis is unusual but occurs with epitheloid sarcoma, synovial sarcoma, rhabdomysosarcoma, angiosarcoma and clear cell sarcoma. Nodal enlargement can also be a reactive response to a recent incisional biopsy.[2] General examination should include a search for café-au-lait patches and other malignancies including breast, thyroid and prostate. Evidence of systemic dissemination, especially to lungs, should be looked for.

Key point 2

- Most soft tissue sarcomas present with a painless gradually increasing mass.

PATHOLOGY

The World Health Organization has defined 50 tumour subtypes of soft tissue sarcomas.[7] These have been classified according to the predominant type of cellular differentiation such as skeletal muscle (rhabdomyosarcoma), fat (liposarcoma), blood vessels (angiosarcoma) or fibrous tissue (fibrosarcoma). There is no evidence to support the concept of a primitive mesenchymal stem cell being the precursor of these tumours. It is more likely that switching-on a given set of genes that programme mesenchymal differentiation in any type of mesenchymal cell may give rise to any mesenchymal neoplasm.[7] Evidence from micro-array and gene chip data suggests that many histological types of soft tissue sarcomas have characteristic patterns of gene expression associated with the process of neoplasia.[4] It is important to determine the histological type of sarcoma as it is an important determinant of prognosis and predictor of clinical behaviour. Leiomyosarcomas and malignant peripheral nerve sheath tumours have a poor prognosis.[8] There are five histological subtypes of liposarcomas (well-differentiated, de-differentiated, myxoid, round cell and pleomorphic) having distinctly different biological behaviour.[7] Immunohisto-chemistry, electron microscopy and cytogenetics may help in identifying the cell type and histological sub-typing of soft tissue sarcomas. The most common histopathological subtypes are malignant fibrous histiocytoma, liposarcoma, synovial sarcoma, leiomyosarcoma and fibrosarcoma.[8] Even with all diagnostic aids, 5–10% of soft tissue sarcomas remain unclassifiable in specialist centres.

Histological grading of soft tissue sarcomas is an important prognostic factor and the TNM staging classification clearly reflects this.[9] Several grading systems have been reported using 3 or 4 grades;[10] however, the TNM staging system utilises a 2-grade classification. Histological grading is based on tumour histological type/subtype, mitoses per high-power field, presence of necrosis, cellular and nuclear morphology and degree of cellularity. The histological grade reflects metastatic potential better than the cellular classification.[10] Most therapeutic decisions are based on the grade of soft tissue sarcomas; therefore, it is important that there is a careful review by the pathologist. Since a high level of discordance can be seen in pathological grading, review by the treating institution is advisable. Pathologists with expertise in sarcomas having access to optimal cytogenetic and molecular diagnostic techniques may be needed to identify and grade soft tissue sarcomas.

INVESTIGATIONS

IMAGING

Imaging studies for soft tissue sarcomas involve evaluation of both the primary lesion and the potential sites of metastasis. Plain radiographs of the extremity are of limited value but may be useful to rule out a primary bone neoplasm and detect calcification characteristic of soft tissue osteosarcoma and synovial sarcoma. They can also show involvement of bone. With the establishment of limb-sparing surgery for soft tissue sarcomas, pre-operative planning is of utmost importance and imaging by computed tomography (CT) or magnetic resonance imaging (MRI) is mandatory. MRI is generally considered the modality of choice for soft tissue sarcomas. MRI can produce images in any plane or in multiple planes to match better more familiar surgical, anatomical or conventional orientations.[11] MRI or contrast-enhanced CT help in demonstrating the relationship of soft tissue sarcomas to the fascia, bones, joints, nerves and major blood vessels. Angiography is seldom necessary. Though MRI is more popular than CT, and is the prevailing modality of choice, it has not shown any statistical advantage over CT in determining tumour involvement of muscle, bone, joint and neurovascular structures.[11,12] Contrast-enhanced CT may be a suitable alternative in situations where MRI is not available or is contra-indicated. Well-differentiated liposarcomas which contain more gross fat can be identified on CT or MRI. Advances in CT and MRI imaging now permit faster acquisition of images and better spatial resolution. Dynamic gadolinium-enhanced MRI can be helpful in distinguishing tumour from oedema. Magnetic resonance spectroscopy may be useful in assessing response to preoperative chemotherapy.[3]

Positron emission tomography (PET) uses [^{18}F]-fluorodeoxyglucose (FDG) to measure tumour glucose uptake as a marker of tumour activity and can be used to quantify tumour activity as opposed to anatomical detail offered by CT and MRI.[13] Several investigators have found that FDG uptake correlates with tumour grade, mitotic rate, cellularity and survival.[14] It has also been used to assess response to neo-adjuvant chemotherapy. Soft tissue sarcomas may show a static tumour response or a very slow reduction in size, especially in myxoid areas. Newer therapies directed at specific molecular targets may be cytostatic and result in tumour growth arrest, which may indicate effective therapy for a patient, as opposed to direct cell-killing mechanisms and tumour shrinkage.[14] Imaging by PET would be especially useful in these situations. PET has also been used to find occult metastatic disease and is being investigated for targeting appropriate biopsy sites in soft tissue sarcomas. A large prospective study is underway to study the value of FDG-PET scan combined with CT scan in predicting disease-free survival in patients receiving neo-adjuvant chemotherapy for soft tissue sarcomas.[15] Currently, as in many other cancers, there is no standard role for PET in screening, diagnosis or staging of soft tissue sarcomas.

Lung is the commonest site of metastasis in patients with extremity soft tissue sarcomas. A chest radiograph is essential though a pre-operative CT of the thorax is preferable for detecting metastasis. Patients with high-grade tumours, 5 cm or larger in size, should undergo more intensive screening for pulmonary metastasis by a chest CT.[16] All patients with an abnormal chest radiograph should also have a chest CT. Extremity myxoid liposarcomas larger than 5 cm have a tendency to metastasise to extrapulmonary soft tissue sites including retroperitoneum and mesentery; therefore, patients should undergo an abdominal and pelvic CT scan.[17] Extremity leiomyosarcoma, epitheloid sarcoma and angiosarcoma should also be considered for an abdominal and pelvic CT scan.[17] Isotope bone scan is not routinely indicated. It is performed only in patients who are symptomatic.

Key point 3

- Magnetic resonance imaging (MRI) is the modality of choice for imaging soft tissue sarcomas. Where MRI is contra-indicated or not available, contrast-enhanced computed tomography is a suitable alternative.

BIOPSY

Any soft tissue mass in an adult that is asymptomatic or is enlarging, is larger than 5 cm, or persists beyond 4–6 weeks should undergo biopsy. The preferred biopsy approach is generally the least invasive technique that enables definitive histological diagnosis and assessment of grade. Biopsy can be performed by fine needle aspiration, core needle biopsy, incisional biopsy or excisional biopsy. Ideally, the clinician who will undertake the definitive treatment should perform the biopsy.[18]

A core needle biopsy is a safe, accurate and economical procedure for diagnosing soft tissue sarcomas.[4,19] It is possible to obtain several cores, possibly from different sites to ensure that the biopsies are representative. Enough tissue is usually obtained for use in several diagnostic tests such as electron microscopy, cytogenetic analysis and flow cytometry. The subtype and grade of the tumour can be determined in 80% of core needle biopsies, and pathologists experienced in examining soft tissue sarcomas have a diagnostic accuracy of 95–99%.[3] The biopsy of superficial lesions is guided by direct palpation; in less accessible soft tissue sarcomas or in tumours with significant

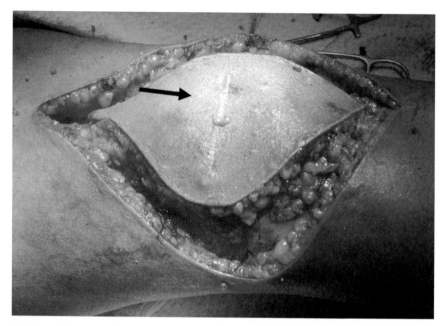

Fig. 2 An ill-placed transverse biopsy scar on thigh requiring extensive skin excision.

amount of necrosis, CT or sonography guided core biopsy can be done. Fine needle aspiration cytology (FNAC) is usually used for the diagnosis of suspected recurrent sarcoma and nodal metastasis where there is an established prior diagnosis and classification of soft tissue sarcomas.[2] It is usually not used for the primary diagnosis of soft tissue sarcomas. However, some authors have argued that FNAC is sufficient to diagnose primary soft tissue sarcomas.[4] The limitations of FNAC are small material yield, difficulty in grading of soft tissue sarcomas, and its dependence on the experience and skills of the cytopathologist. The diagnostic accuracy of FNAC is 60–96%.[20] Core biopsy, however, remains the preferred method for the definitive diagnosis of soft tissue sarcomas.[4,19]

An open biopsy is required when a definitive diagnosis cannot be achieved by core biopsy or FNAC. Open biopsies have a high risk of complications but a small likelihood of a misdiagnosis.[21] Several technical points merit comment. The biopsy incision should be oriented longitudinally along the extremity over its most superficial part to facilitate a subsequent wide local excision that encompasses the biopsy site scar and tumour *en bloc*. The surgeon should avoid raising skin flaps, achieve meticulous haemostasis and dissect through a muscle avoiding inter-muscular or neurovascular planes. Drains, if needed, should be brought out close to the biopsy incision.[22] Excisional biopsy specimens should be properly oriented when being sent to the pathologist. The main pitfalls of biopsy are inappropriate incisions that preclude limb salvage surgery, local spread of tumour to surrounding areas and obtaining inadequate tissue for diagnosis.[23] An ill-placed incision (transverse incision; Fig. 2) may make definitive resection of soft tissue sarcomas more difficult, possibly requiring more extensive soft tissue reconstruction for wound closure and thus needing more extensive postoperative radiation fields to encompass all tissue at risk. An excisional biopsy is usually not done, except for small (usually smaller than 3 cm), subcutaneous tumours, in which a wider re-excision (if needed) is normally straightforward. Any lesion deep to the fascia or lying adjacent to critical structures such as nerves, vessels or bone should undergo an incisional biopsy only.

Key point 4

- Biopsy should establish grade and histological subtype. A core needle biopsy (trucut needle biopsy) provides adequate tissue for histopathological diagnosis. Incisional biopsy, if needed, should be done with great care observing all precautions.

STAGING

The International Union Against Cancer (UICC) and American Joint Committee on Cancer (AJCC) staging system (UICC/AJCC 2002) is currently followed.[9] It is based on the histological grade, tumour size and depth, and the presence of distant or nodal metastasis. Histological grade, depth and tumour size are the primary determinants of UICC/AJCC staging. Soft tissue sarcomas above the superficial investing fascia of the extremity or trunk are designated by the addition of an 'a' in the T-score, whereas tumours invading the fascia or deep to it are designated by a 'b' in the T-score.

MANAGEMENT

The current management of soft tissue sarcomas is by multimodality treatment. Surgery remains the principal therapeutic modality in soft tissue sarcomas. The optimum combination of radiation and chemotherapy with surgery remains controversial.[23]

Key point 5

- The current management of soft tissue sarcomas is multidisciplinary treatment.

SURGERY

Surgical resection is the mainstay of treatment for extremity soft tissue sarcomas. Over the past three decades, there has been a marked decline in the rate of amputations as the primary treatment for extremity soft tissue sarcomas. There is clear evidence that, in patients for whom limb-sparing surgery is an option, a multimodality approach employing limb-sparing surgery combined with pre- or postoperative radiation yields disease-related survival rates comparable to those of amputation while preserving a functional extremity.[24] Soft tissue sarcomas grow in a centrifugal fashion, gradually expanding the surrounding tissue. This leads to the development of a pseudocapsule. Surrounding the pseudocapsule is a reactive zone, which contains small nests of viable, malignant cells that are separate from the tumour itself.

The aim of surgery is to remove the tumour with as wide a margin of normal tissue as possible, while at the same time preserving function of the extremity. Enneking *et al.*[25] classified surgical margins in sarcomas. If the excision passes through the lesion leaving gross tumour behind, it is defined as intra-lesional. If it passes through the reactive zone, it is defined as marginal excision. If the reactive zone is removed intact, with a cuff of normal tissue completely surrounding the lesion, the excision is deemed to be wide. An excision that removes the entire anatomical compartment is a radical excision.

Intralesional excisions (shelling-out procedures) have a nearly 100% local recurrence rate and should not be done. The preferred excision margin for a soft tissue sarcomas is a wide margin. This will remove all of the tumour and the reactive zone, which contains nests of independent, viable, tumour cells. There are no randomised trials to address what constitutes a satisfactory gross resection margin. In general, a margin of 2–3 cm of normal tissue is required for a wide margin, except in the immediate vicinity of functionally important neurovascular structures. Here, in the absence of frank tumour involvement, dissection in the immediate perineural or perivascular plane is performed.

If major vessels are encased, they should be resected and reconstructed as required.[26] It is unusual for soft tissue sarcomas to invade the bone directly. Composite bone and soft tissue resections are indicated primarily for frank bone invasion. In the absence of this, the periosteum is an adequate surgical margin for soft tissue sarcomas treated with wide excision and radiation.[27] If cortical bone is invaded, resection of the bone with reconstruction should be done using a bone graft or an internal prosthesis.[28]

Skin is rarely involved in soft tissue sarcomas and can usually be preserved. Skin and soft tissue reconstruction is required in 10–20% of patients and can reduce complications or prevent amputation.[29] Skin cover may be needed after resection of soft tissue sarcomas in patients with poor biopsy scars, fungating tumours, recurrent soft tissue sarcomas and following pre-operative radiation. Rotational, myocutaneous or fasciocutaneous flaps are commonly used; however, at times, free tissue transfer is needed to cover the defect.[30,31] Difficulties should be anticipated, such as the need for vascular reconstruction or soft tissue coverage of the defect and pre-operative consultation with vascular or plastic surgeons should be sought if their expertise appears necessary during the surgical procedure.

Wide local excision alone is associated with local recurrence in 12–31% of patients.[32–35] Surgical margin of greater than 1 cm is associated with a significantly higher 10-year local control rate compared with margins less than 1 cm.[34]

Surgery alone may be appropriate treatment in selected patients with a favourable prognosis. There are no randomised trials to define specifically these subsets of patients who do not need adjuvant radiotherapy. Based on retrospective studies and few prospective studies, local control rates of 90% or more are achievable in these patients.[34–37] Patients who might reasonably be considered for treatment by surgery alone include those with T1a disease and when microscopic surgical margins are unequivocally negative or preferably wide (1–2 cm tumour-free margin or margin containing an intervening undisturbed fascial plane).[37,38]

Limb-salvage surgery has become the standard of care for extremity soft tissue sarcomas. There is little point in undertaking the risks of limb salvage if a functionless extremity results or if the patient is significantly more likely to be at risk for local recurrence. Local recurrence rates, with proper patient selection and multimodality treatment, are acceptable and range between 5–10%.[16,39,40] The anatomical requirements for extremity function depend on the site of the tumour. In the upper extremity, prosthesis provides poor function; in the distal lower extremity, below-knee amputation and prosthesis may provide better function than a preserved limb damaged by extensive surgery and radiation. In the lower extremity, resection of the sciatic or peroneal nerve can be tolerated with moderate reduction of function.[41] The decision whether to proceed with limb preservation or amputate requires considerable experience on the functional outcomes of various amputation levels.[22]

Amputations are needed in 5–10% of patients and are an important part of local therapy in patients with extremity soft tissue sarcomas. They may be indicated where it is otherwise impossible to achieve adequate tumour-free surgical margins because the lesion involves major neurovascular structures or multiple compartments. Amputations may also be needed for multiple recurrent disease, soft tissue defects which cannot be reconstructed or expected poor limb function with limb salvage.[42]

Key points 6
- Wide margin, function preserving (attempting limb salvage), surgical resection of the tumour is the mainstay of treatment. Amputation is needed in less than 5% of patients.

RADIOTHERAPY

Radiotherapy is an important part of treatment of soft tissue sarcomas where limb salvage is being planned.[43,44] Radiation can be administered pre- or postoperatively by either external beam or by interstitial techniques (brachytherapy). The addition of radiotherapy to limb-sparing surgery produces local control rates of more than 85%.[32,33] This local benefit is without improvement in patient survival.[16] Radiotherapy is indicated for tumours >5 cm in size, where the resection margin is close, positive or unknown and in high-grade tumours.[3,45] As mentioned earlier, there is a subset of patients where radiotherapy can be avoided. Considerable attention has been focused on the optimal sequence of surgery and radiotherapy.[23,46] This is because both pre- and postoperative radiation have specific advantages and disadvantages (Table 1). Pre-operative radiotherapy is usually administered using a total dose

Table 1 Advantages and disadvantages of pre- and postoperative radiation therapy for soft tissue sarcoma

	Advantage	Disadvantage
Pre-operative radiation	• Lower radiation dose (50 Gy) • Smaller treatment volume • Reduced risk for significant fibrosis and oedema	• Greater risk of major wound complications (30%)
Postoperative radiation	• Lower risk for major wound complications (15%)	• Higher radiation dose (66 Gy) • Larger treatment volume • Increased risk for significant fibrosis and oedema

of 50 Gy in 25 × 2-Gy daily fractions and a smaller treatment volume than postoperative radiotherapy. Surgical resection is done 4–6 weeks after completion of radiotherapy. Postoperative radiotherapy is started approximately 4–6 weeks after surgical removal of the tumour and encompasses the entire surgical scar and drain sites.

A randomised clinical trial has evaluated pre-operative versus postoperative radiotherapy in soft tissue sarcomas of limbs.[47] Patients were randomised to pre-operative radiotherapy (50 Gy) and surgery versus surgery followed by postoperative radiotherapy (66 Gy). Increased wound complications requiring invasive wound care and second operative procedures were seen in the pre-operative radiation group (severe wound complication 35% pre-operative radiotherapy versus 17% postoperative radiotherapy). Wound complications with pre-operative radiotherapy occurred much more frequently in patients with lower extremity soft tissue sarcomas (43%) than in patients with upper extremity soft tissue sarcomas (5%). Patients with radiation to the thigh had the highest complication rates (45% pre-operative radiotherapy and 28% postoperative radiotherapy). Though there was slight, but statistically significant, improvement in overall survival in the pre-operative radiation group, the study was not designed to compare survival. It was concluded, from this study, that pre-operative external beam radiation therapy is effective. However, patients should be informed of increased risk for major wound complications, particularly in those with soft tissue sarcomas in the lower extremity. Anatomical site and size of tumour should thus play a role in deciding timing of radiotherapy.

Radiation can be delivered by external beam radiotherapy (EBRT) or brachytherapy. There has been no direct comparison of EBRT to brachytherapy. Brachytherapy involves the insertion of radioactive wires (Iridium-192) into surgically placed catheters traversing the tumour bed. Where the necessary expertise is available for brachytherapy, this technique provides an excellent, cost-effective alternative for appropriate patients with high-grade lesions.[32] Brachytherapy should not be used for patients with low-grade soft tissue sarcomas which are better treated with EBRT.[32,33] Brachytherapy can also be used following surgery for recurrent soft tissue sarcomas previously treated with EBRT.[48] Combination of brachytherapy and EBRT has also been evaluated and has shown an improvement in local control.[49]

Pre-operative radiotherapy may be considered in soft tissue sarcomas with borderline resectability where limb-conserving surgery might become feasible following pre-operative radiotherapy. The benefit has to be weighed against the increased risk of postoperative morbidity. Radiotherapy alone is considered when surgery is inappropriate or is declined by the patient. It achieves local control in 30–60% of patients. Intensity modulated radiotherapy (IMRT) for soft tissue sarcomas is promising, but still investigational.[22]

In patients with unplanned positive surgical margins, radiotherapy does not help in local control. These patients should undergo a re-excision followed by postoperative radiotherapy.[50] In contrast, leaving a carefully considered positive margin adjacent to a critical structure to facilitate limb preservation results in local recurrences rates of less than 10% when planned radiotherapy is carried out.[51]

Key point 7

- Radiation can be given either before or after surgery. Pre-operative radiation has a high incidence of wound complications. Combination of surgery and radiation results in local control in over 85% of patients.

CHEMOTHERAPY

Chemotherapy for soft tissue sarcomas has been used in the adjuvant, neo-adjuvant and palliative settings.[52]

Neo-adjuvant chemotherapy

In the neo-adjuvant (primary or induction chemotherapy) application, it has been used both as single modality (chemotherapy alone) and concurrently with radiation (chemoradiotherapy). Though there are several, strong, theoretical, potential benefits for the use of neo-adjuvant treatment, improved limb salvage and resectability in borderline tumours are the most important for extremity soft tissue sarcomas. The potential disadvantage of response not actually translating into limb conservation and the possibility of tumour progression are major deterrents to neo-adjuvant treatment.

A recently published, retrospective, cohort analysis of neo-adjuvant chemotherapy for primary high grade extremity soft tissue sarcoma has shown that pre-operative chemotherapy with AIM (Doxorubicin/Ifosfamide/Mesna) was associated with a significant improvement in 3-year disease-specific survival (83% versus 62%).[53] However, given the limitations of any retrospective analysis, it is difficult to make any definite recommendations.

The extent of pathological necrosis may be considered a surrogate end-point for survival outcomes in patients with soft tissue sarcomas. Patients with complete pathological necrosis may have improved survival. However, the way in which a response (pathological necrosis) to neo-adjuvant chemotherapy translates into other clinically meaningful outcomes (*e.g.* reduction in scope of surgical resection) is not well defined. Results from the

MD Anderson Cancer Center have shown that pre-operative chemotherapy resulted in a decrease of anticipated surgery in 13% of patients and increase in 9% of patients due to progression.[54] There is, at present, no definite evidence to support the perception that locally advanced soft tissue sarcomas in an extremity can be down-staged enough by induction chemotherapy to permit function preserving limb conserving surgery.[55]

An EORTC Phase II study of neo-adjuvant chemotherapy for 'high-risk' adult soft tissue sarcomas randomised subjects to pre-operative chemotherapy with Doxorubicin and Ifosfamide (3 cycles) followed by conservational surgery and adjuvant radiotherapy versus no pre-operative chemotherapy.[56] It was concluded that this chemotherapy schedule was feasible and did not compromise further surgery and radiation. Although not powered to draw definite conclusions on benefit, no statistically significant survival benefit (DFS or OS) was seen at median follow-up of 7.3 years.

Neo-adjuvant chemoradiation

Several Phase I and II studies have reported favourable results using concurrent chemoradiation for extremity soft tissue sarcomas.[52] A recent Phase II multicentre study of neo-adjuvant chemotherapy and radiation therapy in high-risk, high-grade soft tissue sarcomas of extremities and body wall conducted in the Radiation Therapy Oncology Group (RTOG) trial showed an estimated 3-year rate of disease-free, distant disease-free and overall survival of 56.6%, 64.5% and 75.1%, respectively.[57] However, major toxicity (5% grade 5 (3 deaths) and 83% grade 4) was experienced by the 66 patients enrolled in the study. Given the substantial toxicities of chemoradiation and the open question of whether it provides a durable, overall, survival benefit, it is difficult to make a compelling case for routine administration of neo-adjuvant chemoradiation protocols similar to the RTOG study.

The current NCCN Guideline[17] recommends use of neo-adjuvant therapy (pre-operative RT/CT/CT&RT) for large, high-grade, extremity sarcomas (> 10 cm) at high risk for local recurrences and metastases. Pre-operative chemotherapy or chemoradiation is used in many centres for high-grade tumours to down-stage a large tumour to enable effective surgical resection, especially in the case of chemosensitive histologies.

Adjuvant chemotherapy

Use of adjuvant chemotherapy in resectable soft tissue sarcomas is controversial.[52] The Sarcoma Meta-analysis Collaboration evaluated the effect of adjuvant chemotherapy on localised resectable soft tissue sarcomas in 1568 patients from 14 trials of doxorubicin-based chemotherapy.[58] At a median follow-up of 9.4 years, the time to local and distant recurrence and recurrence-free survival rates were significantly better in the patients who received doxorubicin-based chemotherapy than in the control group. However, the difference in the overall survival rate in the treatment groups was only 4% (P = 0.12). A subset analysis of 886 patients with extremity tumours showed a 7% benefit in survival (P = 0.029).[58] The Italian randomised controlled trial of 104 patients with high-risk primary and locally recurrent extremity and limb girdle soft tissue sarcomas showed a significant difference in overall survival (75 months versus 46 months; P = 0.03) for those given adjuvant chemotherapy.[59]

Subsequently, two other randomised controlled trials of anthracycline/Ifosfamide combination in a relatively small number of patients have shown improvements in 5-year overall survival which are not statistically significant.[60,61] A cohort analysis of patients with localised high-risk extremity soft tissue sarcomas from Memorial Sloan Kettering Cancer Center (New York, USA) and the MD Anderson Cancer Center (Texas, USA) has recently been published.[62] The results of this study have cautioned the interpretation of the randomised trials of adjuvant chemotherapy as the clinical benefits associated with doxorubicin-based chemotherapy in this group of high-risk extremity soft tissue sarcomas are not sustained beyond 1 year. The role of adjuvant chemotherapy in chemosensitive subtypes of soft tissue sarcomas has not been adequately studied. A recent report by Eilber *et al.*[63] has shown improved disease-specific survival in patients with synovial sarcoma of the extremities.

Palliative chemotherapy

The most active chemotherapeutic agents in soft tissue sarcomas are Doxorubicin, Ifosfamide and Dacarbazine (DTIC).Combination chemotherapy is associated with a higher response rate. The most commonly used regimens are MAID (Mesna, Doxorubicin, Ifosfamide, Dacarbazine) and AIM (Doxorubicin, Ifosfamide, Mesna). The role of high-dose chemotherapy with or without autologous bone marrow transplant is not well defined.[4,52,64]

Chemotherapy has been shown to be especially beneficial for certain histopathological subtype of soft tissue sarcomas like synovial sarcoma and myxoid liposarcoma. However, given the limitations of the evidence, where trials have included a mixed heterogeneous group of several subtypes of soft tissue sarcomas, it is difficult to tease out these effects.

Key point 8

- Anthracycline-based postoperative chemotherapy may improve disease-free survival in selected patients who are at high risk of recurrence.

RECURRENT SOFT TISSUE SARCOMA

The management of recurrent soft tissue sarcomas encompasses a hetero-geneous group of patients and clinical scenarios. Locally recurrent soft tissue sarcomas which are resectable and where limb salvage is feasible, should undergo limb salvage. Patients in whom limb salvage is not possible should undergo an amputation.[17,42]

Key point 9

- Patients with local recurrence are treated using the same guidelines as for patients with a new primary lesion.

UNRESECTABLE AND METASTATIC SOFT TISSUE SARCOMAS

In patients with recurrent, locally advanced, soft tissue sarcomas, induction chemotherapy usually does not allow sufficient size reduction to permit limb-preserving surgery.[54] Isolated limb perfusion has been employed in Europe as a limb-sparing treatment for unresectable intermediate or high-grade extremity soft tissue sarcomas.[52] Melphlan in combination with tumour necrosis factor-α (TNF-α) has a better response and limb salvage rate compared to melphlan alone.[17,52] This combination of melphlan and TNF-α is approved in Europe for isolated limb perfusion in patients with locally advanced, high-grade, soft tissue sarcomas of extremities.

In patients presenting with metastases, it is important to distinguish between widely disseminated metastases and limited metastases confined to a single organ. For patients presenting with disseminated disease, the treatment is palliative. Usually these patients receive palliative chemotherapy. In contrast, patients who present with limited metastasis confined to a single organ and limited tumour bulk are treated with a combination of chemotherapy, surgery and radiotherapy. Patients with initial regional nodal involvement may benefit more from nodal dissection compared to those presenting with nodal metastasis after initial treatment of primary soft tissue sarcomas.[65] Despite the poor prognosis associated with metastatic adult soft tissue sarcomas, selected patients with limited pulmonary metastasis undergoing resection of metastatic disease have been shown to have a survival of 22–36% at 5 years.[66]

Key points 10 and 11

- Patients with disseminated metastatic disease are treated with palliative chemotherapy.
- Selected patients with limited metastasis confined to a single organ and limited tumour bulk or regional nodal involvement may benefit from surgical resection (metastasectomy or regional node dissection).

PROGNOSTIC FACTORS

Age (over 60 years), grade, size and stage are important prognostic factors in adult soft tissue sarcomas.[4] However, the most important prognostic variable may be the type and quality of treatment. The 5-year survival rates for stage I, II, III and IV are approximately 90%, 70%, 50% and 10–20%, respectively.[3]

FUTURE DIRECTIONS

New opportunities for improving the therapeutic ratio for patients with soft tissue sarcomas have recently been developed.[67] These include new anti-cancer drugs (e.g. Trabectidin), molecularly targeted therapies (e.g. anti-angiogenic agents, tyrosine kinase inhibitors and mammalian target of rapamycin [mTOR] inhibitors) and gene therapy.[3,64,67,68]

Meaningful progress in soft tissue sarcomas therapy can come only with collaboration, as single institution studies have difficulty in recruiting sufficient number of patients. This will also allow histology specific trials focused on individual tumour types. New chemotherapeutic and biological agents will also bring about new ways of targeting therapy for soft tissue sarcomas.

Key points for clinical practice

- Soft tissue sarcomas are a diverse group of malignant tumours with different biological behaviours.

- Most soft tissue sarcomas present with a painless gradually increasing mass.

- Magnetic resonance imaging (MRI) is the modality of choice for imaging soft tissue sarcomas. Where MRI is contra-indicated or not available, contrast-enhanced computed tomography is a suitable alternative.

- Biopsy should establish grade and histological subtype. A core needle biopsy (trucut needle biopsy) provides adequate tissue for histopathological diagnosis. Incisional biopsy, if needed, should be done with great care observing all precautions.

- The current management of soft tissue sarcomas is multidisciplinary treatment.

- Wide margin, function preserving (attempting limb salvage), surgical resection of the tumour is the mainstay of treatment. Amputation is needed in less than 5% of patients.

- Radiation can be given either before or after surgery. Pre-operative radiation has a high incidence of wound complications. Combination of surgery and radiation results in local control in over 85% of patients.

- Anthracycline-based postoperative chemotherapy may improve disease-free survival in selected patients who are at high risk of recurrence.

- Patients with local recurrence are treated using the same guidelines as for patients with a new primary lesion.

- Patients with disseminated metastatic disease are treated with palliative chemotherapy.

- Selected patients with limited metastasis confined to a single organ and limited tumour bulk or regional nodal involvement may benefit from surgical resection (metastasectomy or regional node dissection).

References

1. Jemal A, Siegel R, Ward E, Murray T, Xu J, Thun MJ. Cancer statistics, 2007. *CA Cancer J Clin* 2007; **57**: 43–66.
2. Ball ABS, Thomas JM. Soft-tissue sarcoma of the limbs and limb girdles. In: Johnson CD,

Taylor I. (eds) *Recent Advances in Surgery*, vol. 15. Edinburgh: Churchill Livingstone, 1992; 69–85.

3. Clark MA, Fisher C, Judson I, Thomas JM. Soft-tissue sarcomas in adults. *N Engl J Med* 2005; **353**: 701–711.

4. Brennan MF, Singer S, Maki RG, O'Sullivan B. Soft tissue sarcoma. In: DeVita VT, Lawrence TS, Rosenberg SA. (eds) *Cancer Principles and Practice of Oncology*, 8th edn. Philadelphia, PA: Lippincott Williams & Wilkins, 2008; 1741–1794.

5. Mannan K, Briggs TW. Soft tissue tumours of the extremities. *BMJ* 2005; **331**: 590.

6. Cooper TM, Sheeham M, Collins D, O'Connor TP. Soft tissue sarcoma of the extremity. *Ann R Coll Surg Engl* 1996; **78**: 453–456.

7. Fletcher CDM, Unni KK, Mertens F. (eds) *Pathology and genetics of tumours of soft tissue and bone*. Vol. 5 of World Health Organization classification of tumours. Lyon, France: IARC Press, 2002.

8. Koea JB, Leung D, Lewis JJ, Brennan MF. Histopathologic type: an independent prognostic factor in primary soft tissue sarcoma of the extremity. *Ann Surg Oncol* 2003; **10**: 432–440.

9. Sobin LH, Wittekind Ch. Tumours of bone and soft tissues: soft tissues. In: *TNM Classification of Malignant Tumors*, 6th edn. New York: Wiley–Liss, 2002; 114–118.

10. Coindre JM. Grading of soft tissue sarcomas. *Arch Pathol Lab Med* 2006; **130**: 1448–1453.

11. Tzeng CWD, Smith JK, Heslin MJ. Soft tissue sarcoma: preoperative and postoperative imaging for staging. *Surg Oncol Clin North Am* 2007; **16**: 389–402.

12. Panicek DM, Gatsonis C, Rosenthal DI *et al*. CT and MRI imaging in the local staging of primary malignant musculoskeletal neoplasms: report of the Radiology Diagnostic Oncology Group. *Radiology* 1997; **202**: 237–246.

13. Schuetze SM. Imaging and response in soft tissue sarcomas. *Hematol Oncol Clin North Am* 2005; **19**: 471–487.

14. Eary JF, Conrad EU. PET imaging: update on sarcomas. *Oncology (Williston Park)* 2007; **21**: 249–252.

15. *Study of Fluorodeoxyglucose positron emission tomography/CT imaging in predicting disease–free survival of patients receiving neoadjuvant chemotherapy for soft tissue sarcomas.* Protocol ID: UMN-2005 LS 080 <www.cancer.gov/clinicaltrials>.

16. Scaife CL, Pisters PW. Combined-modality treatment of localized soft tissue sarcomas of the extremities. *Surg Oncol Clin North Am* 2003; **12**: 355–368.

17. National Comprehensive Cancer Network NCCN. *Clinical Practice Guidelines in Oncology Soft Tissue Sarcoma*, version 2. 2008 <www.nccn.org/professionals/physician-gls/PDF/sarcomas.pdf>.

18. Singer S, Demetri GD, Baldini EH, Fletcher CD. Management of soft-tissue sarcomas: an overview and update. *Lancet Oncol* 2000; **1**: 75–85.

19. Delaney TF. Diagnosis of sarcoma by core biopsy. *J Surg Oncol* 2006; **94**: 1–2.

20. de Saint Aubain Somerhausen N, Fletcher CD. Soft-tissue sarcomas: an update. *Eur J Surg Oncol* 1999; **25**: 215–220.

21. Mankin HJ, Mankin CJ, Simon MA. The hazards of the biopsy, revisited. Members of the Musculoskeletal Tumor Society. *J Bone Joint Surg Am* 1996; **78**: 656–663.

22. Clarkson P, Ferguson PC. Management of soft tissue sarcomas of the extremities. *Expert Rev Anticancer Ther* 2004; **4**: 237–246.

23. Khatri VP, Goodnight Jr JE. Extremity soft tissue sarcoma: controversial management issues. *Surg Oncol* 2005; **14**: 1–9.

24. Rosenberg S, Tepper J, Glatstein E *et al*. The treatment of soft-tissue sarcomas of the extremities: prospective randomized evaluations of (1) limb-sparing surgery plus radiation therapy compared with amputation and (2) the role of adjuvant chemotherapy. *Ann Surg* 1982; **196**: 305–315.

25. Enneking WF, Spanier SS, Goodman MA. A system for the surgical staging of musculoskeletal sarcoma. *Clin Orthop* 1980; **153**: 106–120.

26. Adelani MA, Holt G, Dittus R, Passman MA, Schwartz HS. Revascularization after segmental resection of lower extremity soft tissue sarcomas. *J Surg Oncol* 2007; **95**: 455–460.

27. Lin PP, Pino ED, Normand AN *et al*. Periosteal margin of soft-tissue sarcoma. *Cancer* 2007; **109**: 598–602.

28. Ferguson PC, Griffin AM, O'Sullivan B *et al*. Bone invasion in extremity soft-tissue sarcoma. *Cancer* 2006; **106**: 2692–2700.
29. Carlson GW. The evolution of extremity reconstruction of soft tissue sarcoma. *Ann Surg Oncol* 2006; **13**: 610–611.
30. Saint-Cyr M, Langstein HN. Reconstruction of the hand and upper extremity after tumor resection. *J Surg Oncol* 2006; **94**: 490–503.
31. Heller L, Kronowitz SJ. Lower extremity reconstruction. *J Surg Oncol* 2006; **94**: 479–489.
32. Pisters PW, Harrison LB, Leung DH *et al*. Long-term result of a prospective randomized trail of adjuvant brachytherapy in soft tissue sarcoma. *J Clin Oncol* 1996; **14**: 859–868.
33. Yang JC, Chang AE, Baker AR *et al*. A randomized prospective study of the benefit of adjuvant radiation therapy in the treatment of soft tissue sarcomas of the extremity. *J Clin Oncol* 1998; **16**: 197–203.
34. Baldini EH, Goldberg J, Jenner C *et al*. Long-term outcomes after function-sparing surgery without radiotherapy for soft tissue sarcoma of the extremities and trunk. *J Clin Oncol* 1999; **17**: 3252–3259.
35. Fabrizio PL, Stafford SL, Pritchard DJ. Extremity soft-tissue sarcomas selectively treated with surgery alone. *Int J Radiat Oncol Biol Phys* 2000; **48**: 227–232.
36. Pisters PW, Pollock RE, Lewis VO *et al*. Long-term results of prospective trial of surgery alone with selective use of radiation for patients with T1 extremity and trunk soft tissue sarcomas. *Ann Surg* 2007; **246**: 675–681.
37. Pisters PW, O'Sullivan B, Maki RG. Evidence-based recommendations for local therapy for soft tissue sarcomas. *J Clin Oncol* 2007; **25**: 1003–1008.
38. Pisters PW. Treatment of localized soft-tissue sarcoma: lessons learned. *Oncology (Williston Park)* 2007; **21**: 731–732, 735.
39. Karakousis CP, Zografos GC. Radiation therapy for high grade soft tissue sarcomas of the extremities treated with limb-preserving surgery. *Eur J Surg Oncol* 2002; **28**: 431–436.
40. Popov P, Tukiainen E, Asko-Seljaavaara S *et al*. Soft tissue sarcomas of the lower extremity: surgical treatment and outcome. *Eur J Surg Oncol* 2000; **26**: 679–685.
41. Brooks AD, Gold JS, Graham D *et al*. Resection of the sciatic, peroneal, or tibial nerves: assessment of functional status. *Ann Surg Oncol* 2002; **9**: 41–47.
42. Clark MA, Thomas JM. Amputation for soft-tissue sarcoma. *Lancet Oncol* 2003; **4**: 335–342.
43. Strander H, Turesson I, Cavallin-Stahl E. A systematic overview of radiation therapy effects in soft tissue sarcomas. *Acta Oncol* 2003; **42**: 516–531.
44. Habrand JL, Pechoux CL. Radiation therapy in the management of adult soft tissue sarcomas. *Ann Oncol* 2004; **15**: 187–191.
45. Delaney TF, Kepka L, Goldberg SI *et al*. Radiation therapy for control of soft-tissue sarcomas resected with positive margins. *Int J Radiat Oncol Biol Phys* 2007; **67**: 1460–1469.
46. Wolfson AH. Preoperative vs postoperative radiation therapy for extremity soft tissue sarcoma: controversy and present management. *Curr Opin Oncol* 2005; **17**: 357–360.
47. O'Sullivan B, Davis AM, Turcotte R *et al*. Preoperative versus post-operative radiotherapy in soft-tissue sarcoma of the limbs: a randomised trial. *Lancet* 2002; **359**: 2235–2241.
48. Pearlstone DB, Janjan NA, Feig BW *et al*. Re-resection with brachytherapy for locally recurrent soft tissue sarcoma arising in a previously radiated field. *Cancer J Sci Am* 1999; **5**: 26–33.
49. Andrews SF, Anderson PR, Eisenberg BL, Hanlon AL, Pollack A. Soft tissue sarcoma treated with postoperative external beam radiotherapy with and without low-dose-rate brachytherapy. *Int J Radiat Oncol Biol Phys* 2004; **59**: 475–480.
50. Zagars GK, Ballo MT, Pisters PW *et al*. Surgical margins and reresection in the management of patients with soft tissue sarcoma using conservative surgery and radiation therapy. *Cancer* 2003; **97**: 2544–2553.
51. Gerrand CH, Wunder JS, Kandel RA *et al*. Classification of positive margins after resection of soft-tissue sarcoma of the limb predicts the risk of local recurrence. *J Bone Joint Surg Br* 2001; **83**: 1149–1155.
52. Bauer S, Hartmann JT. Locally advanced and metastatic sarcoma (adult type) including gastrointestinal stromal tumors. *Crit Rev Oncol Hematol* 2006; **60**: 112–130.
53. Grobmyer SR, Maki RG, Demetri GD *et al*. Neo-adjuvant chemotherapy for primary

high-grade extremity soft tissue sarcoma. *Ann Oncol* 2004; **15**: 1667–1672.

54. Meric F, Hess KR, Varma DG *et al*. Radiographic response to neoadjuvant chemotherapy as a predictor of local control and survival in soft tissue sarcomas. *Cancer* 2002; **95**: 1120–1126.

55. Cormier JN, Pollock RE. Soft tissue sarcomas. *CA Cancer J Clin* 2004; **54**: 94–109.

56. Gortzak E, Azzarelli A, Buesa J *et al*. A randomized phase II study on neo-adjuvant chemotherapy for 'high-risk' adult soft-tissue sarcoma. *Eur J Cancer* 2001; **37**: 1096–1103.

57. Kraybill WG, Harris J, Spiro IJ *et al*. Phase II study of neoadjuvant chemotherapy and radiation therapy in the management of high-risk, high-grade, soft tissue sarcomas of the extremities and body wall: Radiation Therapy Oncology Group Trial 9514. *J Clin Oncol* 2006; **24**: 619–625.

58. Sarcoma Meta-analysis Collaboration. Adjuvant chemotherapy for localized resectable soft-tissue sarcoma of adults: meta-analysis of individual data. *Lancet* 1997; **350**: 1647–1654.

59. Frustaci S, Gherlinzoni F, De Paoli A *et al*. Adjuvant chemotherapy for adult soft tissue sarcomas of the extremities and girdles: results of the Italian randomized cooperative trial. *J Clin Oncol* 2001; **19**: 1238–1247.

60. Brodowicz T, Schwameis E, Widder J. Intensified adjuvant IFADIC chemotherapy for adult soft tissue sarcoma: a prospective randomized feasibility trial. *Sarcoma* 2000; **4**: 151–160.

61. Petrioli R, Coratti A, Correale P *et al*. Adjuvant epirubicin with or without ifosfamide for adult soft-tissue sarcoma. *Am J Clin Oncol* 2002; **25**: 468–473.

62. Cormier JN, Huang X, Xing Y. Cohort analysis of patients with localized, high-risk, extremity soft tissue sarcoma treated at two cancer centers: chemotherapy-associated outcomes. *J Clin Oncol* 2004; **22**: 4567–4574.

63. Eilber FC, Brennan MF, Eilber FR *et al*. Chemotherapy is associated with improved survival in adult patients with primary extremity synovial sarcoma. *Ann Surg* 2007; **246**: 105–113.

64. Sinkovics JG. Adult human sarcomas. II. Medical oncology. *Expert Rev Anticancer Ther* 2007; **7**: 183–210.

65. Atalay C, Altinok M, Seref B. The impact of lymph node metastases on survival in extremity soft tissue sarcomas. *World J Surg* 2007; **31**: 1433–1437.

66. Rehders A, Hosch SB, Scheunemann P *et al*. Benefit of surgical treatment of lung metastasis in soft tissue sarcoma. *Arch Surg* 2007; **142**: 70–75.

67. Wunder JS, Nielsen TO, Maki RG, O'Sullivan B, Alman BA. Opportunities for improving the therapeutic ratio for patients with sarcoma. *Lancet Oncol* 2007; **8**: 513–524.

68. Tap WD, Federman N, Eilber FC. Targeted therapies for soft-tissue sarcomas. *Expert Rev Anticancer Ther* 2007; **7**: 725–733.

Vasu Karri Barry Powell

5

New approaches to melanoma treatment

EPIDEMIOLOGY

In the UK, melanoma accounts for the majority of skin cancer death and is the third most common cancer amongst 15–39-year-olds. In 2005, 4370 and 5213 cases were diagnosed in men and women, respectively.[1] The incidence rate has increased by 4-fold during the 30 years from 1975 (3.2 to 13.7 per 100,000 UK population). Although the greatest increase was observed in males (2.5 to 13.2 per 100,000 population) and those over the age of 65 years, the age-standardised rate has been consistently higher in females. Incidence is higher in those from higher socio-economic status, but survival worse in those from lower socio-economic status.[2] In view of the current trend, it has been predicted that the incidence of cutaneous melanoma may double over the next 30 years.[3] The highest incidence of melanoma is observed in Australia and New Zealand with a rate of 30–40 per 100,000 population.[4]

The increasing incidence of melanoma in the UK reflects a trend observed in white populations world-wide. Some investigators have argued that this increase represents improved diagnosis rather than an increase in occurrence.[5] However, this is not supported by European mortality data, particularly of elderly men.[6]

The distribution of melanoma on the body is different for males and females. The back of the trunk and legs are the commonest site for males and females, respectively. Melanoma is rare in non-whites and mostly arises in

Vasu Karri BSc(Hons) MRCS MSc
Specialist Registrar in Plastic Surgery, Melanoma Unit, Department of Plastic & Reconstructive Surgery, St George's Hospital NHS Trust, Blackshaw Road, Tooting, London SW17 0QT, UK. E-mail: vasu_karri@hotmail.com

Barry Powell MCh MA FRCS(Ed) FRCSE (for correspondence)
Reader in Plastic Surgery, National Clinical Advisor in Skin Cancer, Head of Melanoma Service, Melanoma Unit, Department of Plastic & Reconstructive Surgery, St George's Hospital NHS Trust, Blackshaw Road, Tooting, London SW17 0QT, UK. E-mail: bpowell@sgul.ac.uk

non-pigmented sites such as palms of the hands, soles of the feet and subungual regions.

Mortality from melanoma has increased in most white populations in the past few decades world-wide.[7] In the UK from 1971 to 2006, the greatest increase was seen in males over the age of 65 years. During this period, female mortality has fallen to below that of males and stabilised from 1990s onwards. Stabilisation of female mortality has also been reported in North America, Australia and Nordic countries.[8] Despite rising incidence, 5-year survival for melanoma has improved. Superior survival has been reported for females but the reasons for this are poorly understood.[9] It may be due to earlier presentation and diagnosis of thinner tumours.

Key points 1–3

- Melanoma is the most common cause of skin cancer death
- The incidence is increasing in both men and women, with the greatest increase in elderly men.
- Survival is generally worse for men than women with the highest mortality in men over the age of 65 years.

GENETICS

Around 1% of UK melanoma patients report a strong family history.[10] A number of genes have been implicated in melanoma and can be broadly divided into high and low penetrance. This division, however, is somewhat artificial and it is more likely that a range of genes exist with varying penetrance.

LOW PENETRANCE GENES

Melanocortin-1 receptor (MC1R) gene is recognised as a low penetrance melanoma susceptibility gene in white populations. Located on the long arm of chromosome 16, it encodes the receptor for α-melanocyte stimulating hormone (α-MSH) and adrenocorticotrophin (ACTH). The receptor is located on the surface of melanocytes and signals the production of the black pigment eumelanin or redder pigment pheomelanin. However, MC1R is highly polymorphic with more than 80 alleles identified. This polymorphism results in differing proportions of eumelanin and pheomelanin being produced. Individuals who predominantly produce the former tend to have dark hair and dark skin that tans easily. Those individuals with variant MC1R produce pheomelanin and tend to have red/blonde hair and light-coloured skin that tans poorly.[11] Individuals with this phenotype are poorly protected from UV radiation and have an increased risk of melanoma. An increased risk of melanoma also exists in those with variant MC1R without the classic red-hair phenotype.[12] It has been postulated that co-inheritance of MR1C polymorphism with other low penetrance genes may be responsible for the cluster of melanoma in some families.

Other pigmentary genes, including occuloalbinism-2, tyrosinase, tyrosinase-related protein-1 and agouti-related protein, have been identified as melanoma-susceptibility genes.[13]

Melanoma may also be associated with the presence of multiple abnormal naevi, known as the familial atypical mole and melanoma (FAAM) phenotype. The genes responsible for this phenotype are suggested to be low-to-medium penetrance for melanoma. Interestingly, studies of FAAM phenotype families indicate there is a lack of concordance between the phenotype and susceptibility to melanoma. Environmental influence or effect of other genes may be the explanation.

HIGH PENETRANCE GENES

Although the vast majority of melanoma is sporadic, certain families appear to be susceptible to melanoma alone. These families are distinct from those with 'family cancer syndromes', in whom there is a predisposition to a variety of cancers, including melanoma. Studies of melanoma-prone families have revealed mutation in CDKN2A is strongly associated with melanoma development. Germline mutations have been identified in 50% of familial melanoma kindreds with three or more affected members.[14] CDKN2A is located on the short arm of chromosome 9 and is a tumour suppressor gene that encodes two distinct proteins – p16 and p14ARF. The former inhibits cell cycle progression whereas the latter promotes apoptosis or cell cycle arrest. Thus, mutation at the CDKN2A locus may affect either p16, p14ARF or both. Possession of the mutated gene has been calculated to confer a life-time melanoma risk of 58%.[15] Co-inheritance of the CDKN2A mutation and MR1C polymorphism further increases the risk of melanoma in melanoma-prone families.

Mutations in CDK4 and BRAF genes have also been identified in melanoma. Mutation of the CDK4 accounts for a few melanoma kindreds world-wide whereas BRAF mutation has been detected in up to 70% of cases.

Key points 4–5

- MC1R gene is a low penetrance melanoma susceptibility gene that may account for the highest proportion of cases in white populations.

- The majority of families with three or more cases of melanoma have a germline mutation of CDKN2A. Members of such families appear to be at risk of melanoma alone and should be referred for genetic counselling.

DERMOSCOPY

Traditional clinical diagnosis of melanoma has an accuracy of 56–80%.[16] Dermoscopy (dermatoscopy, epiluminescence microscopy) is a non-invasive *in vivo* technique that consists of viewing pigmented skin lesions through a hand-held lens. By using a liquid medium (oil, alcohol, or water) between the lens and skin lesion interface, light reflection is eliminated. Simultaneous optical magnification allows visualisation of the epidermis, dermo-epidermal junction and papillary dermis.[17] A number of diagnostic criteria and algorithms for melanoma have been published with varying sensitivity and specificity. Meta-analysis has demonstrated that, for experienced users, dermoscopy is more accurate than clinical diagnosis.[18] Furthermore, it has also been shown that diagnostic accuracy can be improved in the primary care setting following training.[19]

> **Key point 6**
> * Dermoscopy is an adjunctive tool that can aid clinical diagnosis of melanoma.

STAGING OF MELANOMA

The American Joint Committee on Cancer (AJCC) Tumour-Node-Metastasis (TNM) classification is the most commonly used staging system for cutaneous melanoma (Table 1). The AJCC comprises major melanoma centres in the US, Europe, Australia and national cancer co-operative groups.[20] In 2002, a revised staging system was published (*AJCC Cancer Staging Manual*, 6th edn), based on analysis of prognostic factors of 17,600 melanoma patients from 13 cancer centres.[21]

The 7th edition of the *AJCC Cancer Staging Manual* is due to be implemented in January 2010.

A fundamental difference between the 2002 AJCC TNM classification and the previous version is that the former takes into account 'microstaging attributes' of the primary tumour. These include Breslow thickness, Clark's level and ulceration.[22] Breslow thickness is a quantitative measure of the depth of invasion and recognised as the most important histological prognostic parameter.[23,24,25] Tumour thickness (in millimetres) is measured from the top of the granular layer of the epidermis to the deepest placed melanoma cell. If the tumour is ulcerated, measurement is made from the highest to the deepest melanoma cell. Clark's level represents a qualitative measure of the depth of invasion.[26] Level I tumours do not breach the basement membrane (melanoma *in situ*). Level II tumours invade the papillary dermis, whereas level III tumours fill and expand the papillary dermis. Level IV melanomas invade the reticular dermis and further invasion into the subcutaneous tissue is level IV. In the 2002 classification, T category is subdivided at 1.0, 2.0 and 4.0 mm and Clark's level is only applicable to T1 (≤ 1.0 mm) tumours. It is well established that tumour thickness is a more accurate prognostic marker than level of invasion.[27] For the T1 subgroup of tumours, Clark's level does provide additional prognostic information.[28]

Tumour ulceration is recognised by the new classification as the second most important independent predictor of survival. Patients with ulcerated tumours have the same survival rate as those with non-ulcerated tumours in the next higher thickness category.

CLINICAL VERSUS PATHOLOGICAL STAGE GROUPING

Sentinel lymph node biopsy (SLNB) allows clinicians to stage, accurately and pathologically, the regional lymph node basin. Patients who were initially 'node-negative' may, in fact, have clinically undetectable nodal metastases.

Table 1 AJCC 2002 TNM criteria.[22]
[Used with the permission of the American Joint Committee (AJCC), Chicago. Illinois. The original source for this material is the *AJCC Cancer Staging Manual*, Sixth Edition (2002) published by Springer Science and Business Media LLC, www.springerlink.com]

T classification		
	Thickness	**Ulceration status**
T1	≤ 1.0 mm	a – without ulceration and level II/III
		b – with ulceration or level IV/V
T2	1.01–2.0 mm	a – without ulceration
		b – with ulceration
T3	2.01–4.0 mm	a – without ulceration
		b – with ulceration
T4	> 4.01 mm	a – without ulceration
		b – with ulceration
N classification		
	Metastatic nodes (*n*)	**Nodal metastatic mass**
N1	1	a – micrometastasis*
		b – macrometastasis[†]
N2	2 or 3	a – micrometastasis*
		b – macrometastasis[†]
		c – in-transit metastases/satellite(s) without metastatic nodes
N3	4 or more metastatic nodes, or matted nodes, or in-transit metastases/satellite(s) without metastatic node(s)	
M classification		
	Site	**Serum lactate dehydrogenase**
M1a	Distant skin, subcutaneous tissue, or nodal metastases	Normal
M1b	Lung metastases	Normal
M1c	All other visceral metastases	Normal
	Any distant metastases	Elevated

*Micrometastases are diagnosed after SLNB or elective lymphadenectomy.
[†]Macrometastases are defined as clinically detectable nodal metastases confirmed by therapeutic lymphadenectomy or when gross extracapsular spread is evident.
Staging status should be updated following relapse.

This has significant implications for the patient, both in terms of subsequent management and survival. The issue of pathological staging following SLNB is acknowledged by the new AJCC stage groupings, which makes a clear distinction between clinical and pathological staging (Table 2). The former is performed using excision biopsy microstaging information and clinical examination of the regional lymph nodes. Analysis of the AJCC data indicates there is significant survival differences between patients staged clinically and pathologically. For example, 5-year survival of patients with T2a (1.01–2mm, non-ulcerated) melanoma with clinically negative nodes declines by 16–26% when nodal disease is subsequently detected by SLNB.[29]

Key point 7

• Sentinel lymph node biopsy provides key information which is now utilised in the latest American Joint Committee on Cancer (AJCC) pathological stage groupings.

Table 2 AJCC 2002 stage groupings.[22]

[Used with the permission of the American Joint Committee (AJCC), Chicago. Illinois. The original source for this material is the *AJCC Cancer Staging Manual*, Sixth Edition (2002) published by Springer Science and Business Media LLC, www.springerlink.com]

	Tumour (N)	Nodes (N)	Metastases (M)
Clinical staging			
0	Tis	N0	M0
IA	T1a	N0	M0
IB	T1b–T2a	N0	M0
IIA	T2b–T3a	N0	M0
IIB	T3b–T4a	N0	M0
IIC	T4b	N0	M0
III	Any T	Any N	M0
IV	Any T	Any N	M1
Pathological staging			
0	0	N0	M0
IA	T1a	N0	M0
IB	T1b–T2a	N0	M0
IIA	T2b–T3a	N0	M0
IIB	T3b–T4a	N0	M0
IIC	T4b	N0	M0
IIIA	T1–4a	N1a–N2a	M0
IIIB	T1–4b	N1a	M0
	T1–4b	N2a	M0
	T1–4a	N1b	M0
	T1–4a	N2b	M0
	T1–4a	N1c	M0
	T1–4b	N2c	M0
IIIC	T1–4b	N1b	M0
	T1–4b	N2b	M0
	Any T	N3	M0
IV	Any T	Any N	Any M

By convention, clinical staging should be applied after excision biopsy of the primary melanoma and clinical evaluation for metastases.
Pathological staging includes microstaging of the primary melanoma and information derived from SLNB or complete lymphadenectomy.

SENTINEL LYMPH NODE BIOPSY

Staging of the draining nodal basin of a primary melanoma was previously achieved by elective lymph node dissection (ELND). This procedure was limited to high-risk melanoma and associated with a high degree of morbidity. As only 20% of patients with melanoma thicker than 1 mm have lymph node metastases, up to 80% of patients underwent a procedure that provided no benefit. Furthermore, four randomised controlled trials indicated ELND offered no survival advantage.

Sentinel lymph node biopsy (SLNB) described by Morton *et al.*[30] is a minimally invasive procedure that allows staging of the entire lymph node basin. It is based on the premise that metastatic cells migrate from the primary tumour in a sequential manner, travelling via afferent lymphatics to the first 'sentinel' lymph node(s) within a nodal basin. As the sentinel node is the first site where metastatic cells can reside, its tumour status can be considered representative of all nodes in the basin. If pathological examination subsequently reveals micrometastases, completion lymphadenectomy can be offered. Thus, patients who have negative SLNB can be spared completion lymphadenectomy and associated morbidity. Compared with elective lymphadenectomy, SLNB offers similar accuracy at detecting lymph node micrometastases. Furthermore, lower morbidity and cost-saving are recognised advantages. Knowing the disease status of the regional lymph node basin is one of the most important prognostic indicators.

PATIENT SELECTION

The indications for SLNB vary between specialist centres. Patients with melanoma of Breslow thickness 1.0–4.0 mm are considered appropriate candidates. However, SLNB has also been considered appropriate for tumours ≤ 1 mm, if Clark's level III has been reached or 'vertical growth phase' pattern exists.

At the International Sentinel Node Society meeting in February 2008, consensus was reached on the qualifying criteria for melanoma SLNB.[31] These include:

1. Tumour thickness ≥ 1 mm.

2. Tumour thickness < 1 mm, but associated with one or more co-risk factors (ulceration, mitotic activity > 1 and Clark level IV). These risk factors gain significance when tumour thickness is > 0.75 mm, the patient is young, or both.

These indications are only applicable in the presence of clinically normal regional lymph nodes.

TECHNICAL ASPECTS OF SLNB

In our department, SLNB is performed at the time of wide local excision. On the morning of surgery, technetium-99 (^{99}Tc)-labelled microcolloid is injected intradermally at the site of the primary tumour. The volume of microcolloid injected is determined by the size of the scar. Mapping of lymphatic drainage and identification of one or more sentinel nodes is achieved by static and dynamic scintography (Fig. 1). Location of the SLN is marked on the patient's skin and subcutaneous depth recorded. Performing wide local excision prior to SLNB is not recommended as surgery may disrupt lymphatic channels with resultant formation of an aberrant drainage pattern.

The SLN is identified intra-operatively by intradermal injection of Patent Blue dye at the site of the primary tumour. The dye travels in afferent lymphatics to the sentinel node of the regional nodal basin. A skin incision is made over the node in a manner that would facilitate re-excision of the scar if completion lymphadenectomy of the basin is undertaken. The SLN is identified by the blue stain and radioactivity count, measured using a hand-held gamma-probe.

The SLN is excised, embedded in paraffin and analysed using haematoxylin and eosin (H&E) staining and immunohistochemistry.

BENEFIT OF SLNB

The Multicenter Selective Lymphadenectomy Trial (MSLT-1) represents the only prospective randomised trial (RCT) that has evaluated the survival benefit of SLNB.[32] Patients with melanoma more than 1 mm were randomly assigned to wide excision plus SLNB (with immediate completion

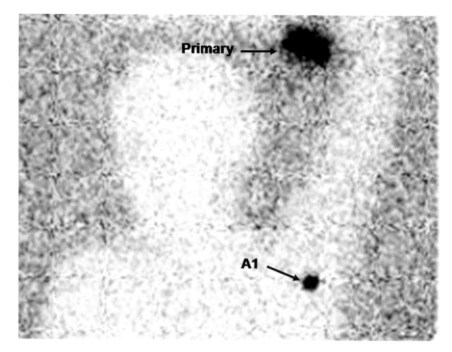

Fig. 1 Lymphoscintography demonstrating a single sentinel node in the left axilla (A1). The primary was on the left forearm.

lymphadenectomy for sentinel node metastases) or wide excision and clinical observation (with completion lymphadenectomy if nodal disease subsequently became evident). The 4th interim analysis presented in February 2008, at median follow-up of 8 years, indicated that SLNB improves disease-free survival but there was no improvement in overall survival. The 5th and final analysis is awaited.

It is clear that SLNB is a minimally invasive staging procedure and most important predictor of overall survival.[33] Data from the AJCC staging database indicate the number of positive lymph nodes is the most important predictor of survival in patients with stage III disease.

SURGICAL TREATMENT

Wide local excision remains the standard of care for primary cutaneous melanoma. The tumour or excision-biopsy scar is excised *en bloc* with a margin

---

Key points 8 and 9

- The tumour status of the sentinel node is considered representative of the entire lymphatic basin.
- Sentinel lymph node biopsy does not improve overall survival but remains the best staging tool and prognostic indicator for overall survival.

Table 3 UK Melanoma Study Group excision margins

Breslow thickness	Excision margin
In situ	5 mm
< 1 mm	1 cm
1–2 mm	1–2 cm
2.1–4.0 mm	2–3 cm[a]
> 4 mm	2–3 cm[b]

For melanoma > 1.5 mm, a 2-cm excision margin is preferred.
[a]A 3-cm margin should be recommended if direct closure can be obtained.
[b]There is no evidence to support using a margin >3 cm.[48]

of normal skin and subcutaneous tissue down to deep fascia. The aim of wide local excision is to reduce the risk of local recurrence.

For many years, wide local excision with a 5-cm margin was the standard. This was derived from the work of Handley who suggested removal of 2 inches of subcutaneous tissue down to the level of muscle fascia, together with a radical removal of lymph nodes.[34] However, during the last two decades a number of studies suggested such an aggressive resection was not necessary.[35,36] Moreover, wider excision may decrease the incidence of local recurrence but not improve survival.[37] Two recent meta-analyses of randomised controlled trials that evaluated wide versus narrow excision margins for trunk or extremity melanoma indicated wide excision offered no benefit over narrow excision.[38,39] Specifically, overall survival, disease-free survival and local recurrence rates were not adversely affected by narrow excision. The current UK Melanoma Study Group margins for excision are given in Table 3.[40] The suggested margins may be adjusted for cosmetic or functional reasons, for example, around the eye.

ADJUVANT THERAPY

Over the past three decades, numerous adjuvant therapies have been evaluated for melanoma. So far, no single agent has significantly improved survival in metastatic disease.

CHEMOTHERAPY

Dacarbazine (DTIC) is commonly used for the treatment of metastatic disease. Partial and complete response rate, however, is limited to 14–20%. Moreover, RCTs have shown DTIC does not impart any survival advantage when compared to supportive care. Combination chemotherapy regimens with DTIC (*e.g.* cisplastin and vincristine) have generated better tumour response rates. However, these polychemotherapy regimens do not improve survival compared with DTIC alone.

VACCINES

There is currently no vaccine that effectively treats advanced melanoma. Non-specific immunostimulant Bacille Calmette-Guérin (BCG) initially showed promise, inducing regression in up to 80% of cutaneous metastases when injected intralesionally. However, subsequent RCTs have not demonstrated a benefit.[41]

Ganglioside GM2-KLH21 vaccine has recently been evaluated in the treatment of stage II melanoma. Gangliosides are unique cell-surface glycolipids that are often over-expressed in melanoma. In a large phase III clinical trial, it was found that adjuvant GM2-KLH21 vaccination was ineffective and could even be detrimental for stage II melanoma patients.[42]

INTERFERONS

The Eastern Cooperative Oncology Group (ECOG) trial is the only study that has demonstrated a benefit with adjuvant therapy for stage III disease. The use of high-dose interferon-α (IFN-α) improved both 5-year disease-free and overall survival.[43] In a recent pooled analysis of the same data, only an improvement in disease-free survival was demonstrated.[44] Use of low dose IFN-α in patients with resected stage III disease, however, does not improve either disease-free or overall survival.[45]

Investigators have also evaluated pegylated interferon (PEG-IFN), an alternative formulation that lasts longer in the body. The results of a recent RCT indicate PEG-IFN increases disease-free survival in patients with stage III melanoma but not overall survival.[46] However, this benefit was only evident for those patients with stage III disease as shown by positive SLNB.

One of the main difficulties with evaluating adjuvant therapies is the inaccuracy of clinical staging of regional lymph nodes. Patients recruited into trials may have microscopic nodal metastases that not palpable. Furthermore, pathological analysis of lymph nodes using current techniques may not detect 'submicroscopic' metastases. With the advent of SLNB and reverse transcriptase polymerase chain reaction (RT-PCR) analysis of lymph nodes, patients can now be more accurately staged. One such study to incorporate these advances is the Sunbelt Melanoma Trial.[47] This RCT compared completion lymphadenectomy and high-dose adjuvant IFN-α with lymphadenectomy alone in patients with positive SLNB. RT-PCR was also used to analyse further negative sentinel lymph nodes and, if positive, those

---

Key points 10–13

- Dacarbazine is the standard chemotherapy agent used for metastatic disease.

- Many vaccines are in advanced stages of development, but no single agent has been shown to be effective against advanced melanoma.

- Adjuvant interferon-α in high-risk melanoma improves disease-free survival.

- Sentinel lymph node biopsy and reverse transcriptase polymerase chain analysis of lymph nodes allows accurate staging of patients. These advances in staging may help identify subgroups of patients who will benefit from future adjuvant therapies.

patients were also included in one arm of the study. The results of the trial were recently published and demonstrate no benefit for adjuvant IFN-α for patients with a single positive sentinel lymph node. Furthermore, patients who had negative SLNB but positive RT-PCR for melanoma cells did not have improved disease-free or overall survival after undergoing lymphadenectomy or lymphadenectomy and IFN-α.

NOVEL APPROACHES

In the search for a novel immunological therapy for melanoma, researchers have focused their attention on T-cell activation and regulation. T-cell activation is a complex process and involves the expression of CTLA-4. This antigen serves to moderate the T-cell response by acting as a negative-feedback 'brake'. Thus, by synthesizing antibodies to CTLA-4, it is hoped that the T-cell response to melanoma cells is promoted. Two human anti-CTLA-4 monoclonal antibodies (Ipilimum and Tremelimumab) are currently being evaluated in clinical trials.

TARGETING SIGNAL TRANSDUCTION PATHWAYS

In melanoma, it is recognised that mutation in B-Raf occurs in 60–70% of melanoma cell lines. The exact role of mutant B-Raf in melanoma tumourgenesis is not known. This protein is integral to signal transduction from the cell membrane to the nucleus. B-Raf mutations have also been detected in non-malignant naevi, suggesting another mechanism is involved for malignant transformation. Currently, one B-Raf inhibitor (BAY 43-9006) is being evaluated in clinical trials of melanoma patients. Unfortunately, results from Phase II trials using BAY 43-9006 as monotherapy against advanced melanoma have been disappointing. Clinical trials are also being conducted investigating BAY 43-9006 in combination with other chemotherapy agents.

Key points 14 and 15

- The B-Raf and Ras signal transduction pathways are potential targets for melanoma treatment.
- BAY 43-9006 is a general Raf inhibitor that is being currently evaluated for advanced melanoma.

CONCLUSIONS

Melanoma is the most common cause of skin cancer death. Surgical excision remains the only effective treatment. During the last 30 years, little progress has been made in the treatment of metastatic disease. Adjuvant therapy for resected regional disease and chemotherapy for metastatic disease impart only a modest improvement in survival. As our understanding of molecular pathways in melanoma improves, alternative therapeutic options may yield success. Early detection is paramount in the successful treatment of melanoma.

Key points for clinical practice

- Melanoma is the most common cause of skin cancer death

- The incidence is increasing in both men and women, with the greatest increase in elderly men.

- Survival is generally worse for men than women with the highest mortality in men over the age of 65 years.

- MC1R gene is a low penetrance melanoma susceptibility gene that may account for the highest proportion of cases in white populations.

- The majority of families with three or more cases of melanoma have a germline mutation of CDKN2A. Members of such families appear to be at risk of melanoma alone and should be referred for genetic counselling.

- Dermoscopy is an adjunctive tool that can aid clinical diagnosis of melanoma.

- Sentinel lymph node biopsy provides key information which is now utilised in the latest American Joint Committee on Cancer (AJCC) pathological stage groupings.

- The tumour status of the sentinel node is considered representative of the entire lymphatic basin.

- Sentinel lymph node biopsy does not improve overall survival but remains the best staging tool and prognostic indicator for overall survival.

- Dacarbazine is the standard chemotherapy agent used for metastatic disease.

- Many vaccines are in advanced stages of development, but no single agent has been shown to be effective against advanced melanoma.

- Adjuvant interferon-α in high-risk melanoma improves disease-free survival.

- Sentinel lymph node biopsy and reverse transcriptase polymerase chain analysis of lymph nodes allows accurate staging of patients. These advances in staging may help identify subgroups of patients who will benefit from future adjuvant therapies.

- The B-Raf and Ras signal transduction pathways are potential targets for melanoma treatment.

- BAY 43-9006 is a general Raf inhibitor that is being currently evaluated for advanced melanoma.

References

1. Cancer Research UK. <www.cancerresearchuk.org> [Accessed 2008].
2. Quinn M, Babb P, Brock A, Kirby L et al. Cancer Trends in England and Wales 1950–1999. London: SMPS Office of National Statistics, 2004; 66.

3. Diffey BL. The future incidence of cutaneous melanoma within the UK. *Br J Dermatol* 2004; **151**: 868–872.
4. Parkin DM Bray F, Ferlay J, Pisani P. Global cancer statistics 2002. *CA Cancer J Clin* 2005; **55**: 74–108.
5. Welch HG, Woloshin S, Schwartz LM. Skin biopsy rates and incidence of melanoma: population-based ecological study. *BMJ* 2005; **331**: 481.
6. De Vries E, Bray F, Coebergh JWW, Parkin DM. Changing epidemiology of malignant cutaneous melanoma in Europe in 1953–1997: rising trends in incidence and mortality but recent stabilisations in Western Europe and decreases in Scandinavia. *Int J Cancer* 2003; **107**: 119–126.
7. Lens MB, Dawes M. Global perspectives of contemporary epidemiological trends of cutaneous malignant melanoma. *Br J Dermatol* 2004; **150**: 179–185.
8. La Vecchia C, Lucchini F, Negri E *et al.* Recent declines in worldwide mortality from cutaneous melanoma in youth and middle age. *Int J Cancer* 1999; **31**: 62–66.
9. Scoggins CR, Ross MI, Reintgen DS *et al.* Gender-related differences in outcome for melanoma patients. *Ann Surg* 2006; **243**: 693–698.
10. Newton JA, Bataille V, Griffiths K *et al.* How common is the atypical mole syndrome phenotype in apparently sporadic melanoma? *J Am Acad Dermatol* 1993; **29**: 989–996.
11. Valverde P, Healy I, Jackson I *et al.* Variants of the melanocyte stimulating hormone receptor gene are associated with red hair and fair skin in humans. *Nat Genet* 1995; **11**: 328–330.
12. Palmer JS, Duffy DL, Box NF *et al.* Melanocortin-1 receptor polymorphisms and risk of melanoma: is the association explained solely by pigmentation phenotype? *Am J Hum Genet* 2000; **66**: 176–186.
13. Jannot AS, Meziani R, Bertrand G *et al.* Allele variations in the OCA2 gene (pink-eyed-dilution locus) are associated with genetic susceptibility to melanoma. *Eur J Hum Genet* 2005; **13**: 913–920.
14. Lesueur F, de Lichy M, Barrois M *et al.* The contribution of large genomic deletions at the CDKN2A locus to the burden of familial melanoma. *Br J Cancer* 2008; **99**: 364–370.
15. Bishop DT, Demenais F, Goldstein AM *et al.* Geographical variation in the penetrance of CDKN2A mutations for melanoma. *J Natl Cancer Inst* 2002; **94**: 894–903.
16. Morton CA, Mackie RM. Clinical accuracy of the diagnosis of cutaneous melanoma. *Br J Dermatol* 1998; **138**: 283–287.
17. Argenziano G, Soyer HP. Dermoscopy of pigmented skin lesions: a valuable tool for early diagnosis of melanoma. *Lancet Oncol* 2001; **2**: 443–449.
18. Kittler H, Pehamberger H, Wolff K *et al.* Diagnostic accuracy of dermoscopy. *Lancet Oncol* 2002; **3**: 159–165.
19. Argenziano G, Puig S, Zalaudek I *et al.* Dermoscopy improves accuracy of primary care physicians to triage lesions suggestive of skin cancer. *J Clin Oncol* 2006; **24**: 1877–1882.
20. Markovic SN, Erickson LA, Rao RD *et al.* Malignant melanoma in the 21st century. Part 2: staging, prognosis and treatment. *Mayo Clin Proc* 2007; **82**: 490–513.
21. Balch CM, Soong SJ, Gershenwald JE *et al.* Prognostic factors analysis of 17,600 melanoma patients: validation of the American Joint Committee on Cancer melanoma staging system. *J Clin Oncol* 2001; **19**: 3622–3634.
22. Greene FL, Page DL, Fleming ID *et al.* Melanoma of the Skin, TNM Definition, Clinical Stage Grouping, Pathologic Stage Grouping. *AJCC Cancer Staging Manual*, 6th edn. New York: Springer, 2002; 211–212
23. Breslow A. Thickness, cross-sectional areas and depth of invasion in the prognosis of cutaneous melanoma. *Ann Surg* 1970; **172**: 902–908.
24. Balch CM, Murad TM, Soong SJ, Ingalls AL, Richards PC, Maddox WA. Tumour thickness as a guide to surgical management of clinical stage 1 melanoma patients. *Cancer* 1979; **43**: 883–888.
25. Clark Jr WH, Elder DE, Guerry IV D *et al.* Model predicting survival in stage 1 melanoma based on tumour progression. *J Natl Cancer Inst* 1989; **81**: 1893–1904.
26. Clark Jr WH, From L, Bernardino EA, Mihm MC. The histogenesis and biologic behaviour of primary human malignant melanomas of the skin. *Cancer Res* 1969; **29**: 705–727.
27. Balch CM, Buzaid AC, Atkins MB *et al.* A new American Joint Committee on Cancer

staging system for cutaneous melanoma. *Cancer* 2000; **88**: 1484–1491.

28. Marghoob AA, Koenig K, Bittencourt FV *et al*. Breslow thickness and Clark level in melanoma: support for including level in pathology reports and in American Joint Committee on Cancer Staging. *Cancer* 2000; **88**: 589–595.

29. Balch CM, Buzaid AC, Soong SJ *et al*. Final version of the American Joint Committee on Cancer staging system for cutaneous melanoma. *J Clin Oncol* 2001; **19**: 3635–3648.

30. Morton DL, Wen DR, Wong JH *et al*. Technical details of intraoperative lymphatic mapping for early stage melanoma. *Arch Surg* 1992; **127**: 392–399.

31. Balch C, Gershenwald JE, Ross MI *et al*. Consensus findings of 6th Biennial Meeting International Sentinel Node Society 2008. *Ann Surg Oncol* 2008; **15 (Suppl 1)**: 1–64.

32. Morton DL, Thompson JF, Cochran AJ *et al*. Sentinel-node biopsy or nodal observation in melanoma. *N Engl J Med* 2006; **355**: 1307–1317.

33. McMasters KM, Noyes RD, Reintgen DS *et al*. Lessons learned from the Sunbelt Melanoma Trial. *J Surg Oncol* 2004; **86**: 212–223.

34. Handley WS. The pathology of melanotic growths in relation to their operative treatment. *Lancet* 1907; **i**: 927–933, 996–1003.

35. Breslow A, Macht SD. Optimal size of resection margins for thin cutaneous melanoma. *Surg Gynecol Obstet* 1977; **145**: 691–692.

36. Olsen G. The malignant melanoma of the skin: new theories based on a study of 500 cases. *Acta Chir Scand* 1966; **365**: 1–222.

37. Ackerman AB, Scheiner AM. How wide and deep is wide and deep enough? A critique of surgical practice in excisions of primary cutaneous malignant melanoma. *Hum Pathol* 1983; **14**: 743–744.

38. Haigh PI, DiFronzo AL, McCready DR. Optimal excision margins for primary cutaneous melanoma: a systematic review and meta-analysis. *Can J Surg* 2003; **46**: 419–426.

39. Lens MB, Nathan P, Bataille V. Excision margins for primary cutaneous melanoma; updated pooled analysis of randomized controlled trials. *Arch Surg* 2007; **142**: 885–891.

40. Roberts DLL, Anstey AV, Barlow RJ *et al*. U.K. guidelines for the management of cutaneous melanoma. *Br J Dermatol* 2002; **146**: 7–17.

41. Sondak VK, Wolfe JA. Adjuvant therapy for melanoma. *Curr Opin Oncol* 1997; **9**: 189–204.

42. Eggermont AM, Suciu S, Ruka W *et al*. EORTC 18961: post-operative adjuvant ganglioside GM2-KLH21 vaccination treatment vs observation in stage II (T3-T4N0M0) melanoma: 2nd interim analysis led to an early disclosure of the results. *J Clin Oncol* 2008; **26**: abstract 9004.

43. Kirkwood JM, Stawderman MH, Ernstoff MS *et al*. Interferon alfa-2b adjuvant therapy of high-risk resected cutaneous melanoma: the Eastern Cooperative Oncology Group trial Est 1684. *J Clin Oncol* 1996; **14**: 7–17.

44. Kirkwood JM, Manola J, Ibrahim J *et al*. A pooled analysis of Eastern Cooperative Oncology Group and intergroup trials of adjuvant high-dose interferon for melanoma. *Clin Cancer Res* 2004; **10**: 1670–1677.

45. Cascinelli N, Belli F, Mackie RM *et al*. Effect of long-term adjuvant therapy with interferon alpha-2a in patients with regional node metastases from cutaneous melanoma: a randomised trial. *Lancet* 2001; **358**: 866–869.

46. Eggermont AM, Suciu S, Santinami M *et al*. Adjuvant therapy with pegylated interferon alfa-2b versus observation alone in resected stage III melanoma: final results of EORTC 18991, a randomised phase III trial. *Lancet* 2008; **372**: 117–126.

47. McMasters KM, Ross MI, Reintgen DS *et al*. Final results of the Sunbelt Melanoma Trial. *J Clin Oncol* 2008; **26**: abstract 9003.

48. Heaton KM, Sussman JJ, Gershenwald JE *et al*. Surgical margins and prognostic factors in patients with thick (> 4 mm) primary melanoma. *Ann Surg Oncol* 1998; **5**: 322–328.

Shirish G. Ambekar Kulvinder S. Lall

6

Update on advances in cardiac surgery

A surgeon who tries to suture a heart wound deserves to lose the esteem of his colleagues.

Theodore Billroth, 1883

Within a few years of this statement, L. Rehn took a stitch on the heart and a new era of cardiac surgery was born. Various wars including World War 1 and World War 2, the Korean War, the Vietnam conflict and the Gulf wars have made surgeons more experienced in treating open cardiac wounds. These wars also gave a major impetus to the advancement of science and technologies in these fields. There has been exponential growth in various fields of cardiac surgery over last 100 years.

ADVANCES IN DIAGNOSIS

New technologies are continuously evolving to aid diagnosis of various pathologies of the heart and in assessing pathophysiological parameters. Oesophageal Doppler and LiDCO (Lithium Dilution Cardiac Output) methods measure stroke volumes, cardiac output and systemic vascular resistance in critically ill patients.[1,2] These are relatively non-invasive methods as against Swan-Ganz catheter monitoring.

Two-dimensional echocardiography (2-D ECHO) has been in practice for many decades now. Its use in assessment of congenital cardiac anomalies, cardiac function, valvular morphology and pathologies (such as pericardial

Shirish G. Ambekar MBBS MS MCh DMS(Greenwich) FRCSEd(CTh) (for correspondence)
Specialist Registrar in Cardiothoracic Surgery, Department of Cardiothoracic Surgery,
St Bartholomew's Hospital, West Smithfield, Whitechapel, London EC1 7BE, UK.
E-mail: shirishambekar@hotmail.com

Kulvinder S. Lall MBBS FRCSEng(CTh)
Consultant Cardiothoracic Surgeon, St Bartholomew's Hospital, West Smithfield, Whitechapel,
London EC1 7BE, UK. E-mail: kulvinder.lall@bartsandthelondon.nhs.uk

diseases) is well known. Transoesophageal echocardiography (TOE) is superior in assessing the above mentioned conditions. The probe sits in the oesophagus right behind the left atrium thereby avoiding artefacts like bone (chest wall) and air (lungs). Recently, three-dimensional echo (3-D ECHO) has been applied in clinical practice. It is clearly superior to the first two modalities of ECHO in assessing cardiac morphology, cardiac volumes and its function. It is used as a teaching and research tool. It excels in diagnosing paravalvular leaks, masses, vegetations and displaying coronary anomalies.[3,4] 3-D ECHO currently is at the beginning of its evolution and other technologies are being incorporated to improve image display and its reconstruction. Stereoscopy, halography and generation of 3-D models will help the perception of cardiac morphology in future.[5]

Intravascular ultrasound (IVUS) helps to delineate intracoronary plaques in a three-dimensional fashion, thus becoming an important complimentary tool to coronary angiography which gives an image in the two dimensional plane. Positron emission tomography (PET) and cardiac magnetic resolution are newer modalities. They are superior in assessing myocardial reversibility and regional wall motion abnormalities. Cardiac magnetic resolution is used to diagnose various congenital anomalies, left ventricle aneurysms, aortic dissections and valvular dysfunctions. Its use is currently limited because of high initial costs of installation. Electron beam computerised tomography (EBCT) is another tool increasingly used in delineating coronary anatomy. It gives significantly low radiation doses and renal dysfunction (due to dye) can be avoided in high-risk patients. As the technology improves, it will have the potential to be used in mass screening for coronary calcification.

Key point 1

- Newer diagnostic modalities have led to early detection and better management of cardiac pathologies.

TECHNICAL ADVANCES

Advances in cardiac surgery would not have been possible without the simultaneous advances in allied fields like cardiac anaesthesia, intensive care management and blood bank. Easy availability of blood and its constituents (*e.g.* FFP, platelets, cryoprecipitate and individual factors like factors VII and VIII) mean that cardiac surgery can be performed with relative ease in challenging situations such as re-do surgery, surgery in haemophiliacs, Jehovah's witnesses, octogenarians and the complex congenital cyanotic conditions.

Control of bleeding is the biggest challenge to any surgeon; however, controlling blood loss from the heart and aorta is critical to the success of cardiac surgery. Today's cardiac surgeon has a battery of products available at his disposal. Tissel, Flo-Seal, Nu-knit, Bio Glue are a few examples. These new products: (i) provide thrombin and fibrinogen to facilitate clotting; (ii) act as a mechanical haemostat by closing needle holes; or (iii) provide a skeleton for the formation of clot. Advances in suture technology have resulted in needles becoming smaller, tougher and atraumatic. Adjuncts like Teflon pledgets, bovine pericardium and Gore-Tex or Dacron patches have all helped in achieving blood-tight vascular anastomoses.

> ## Key point 2
> • Development of anaesthesia, blood bank and critical care manage-
>   ment has helped achieve better results of cardiac surgery.

RISK STRATIFICATION

There are various systems of risk stratification in the practice of medicine and surgery, including PARSONNET, APACHE and BAYES. In cardiac surgery, currently the European System for Cardiac Operative Risk Evaluation (EuroSCORE) is utilised for assessment of the risks and prognosis of the patient undergoing cardiac surgery.[6] Various scores are given to the co-morbid conditions. By adding these numbers, the predicted mortality can be estimated. It is a very simple and fairly accurate system for risk stratification. The system also helps each centre to compare its results nationally; within a centre, different surgeons can be compared on the basis of their individual results. It is also a good teaching and research tool. Over the years, as the mortality of any particular cardiac operation has fallen, it has helped surgeons to take on increasingly complex procedures in challenging scenarios.

ADVANCES IN VALVE TECHNOLOGY

Rapid growth in the fields of biophysics, bioengineering, metallurgy, gene therapy and tissue culture has resulted in the development of valve prostheses, which mimic native human valves (Fig. 1). Laboratories in the developed world have become expert in harvesting, procurement and preservation of homografts. Both autografts and homografts are good prostheses for paediatric cardiac surgical practice. Xenografts have also become more durable (due to use of bovine and equine pericardium).

There is a subset of patients where the risk of aortic valve replacement by conventional open technique is very high due to the presence of life-threatening co-morbidity. In such patients, the aortic valve can be implanted percutaneously. The procedure can be performed antegradely through left ventricle or retrogradely through the aorta. The prosthesis is catheter-mounted and, when the catheter is placed at the optimal position, the valve is opened like an umbrella and sits in its position with the help of a special frame or prongs. This revolutionary technique is still in its infancy and lacks the evidence base for routine use. Currently, two multicentre trials are underway – I-REVIVE in Europe and REVIVAL in the US.

As the pitfalls of valve prosthesis came to light, the focus of treatment for valvular heart disease has shifted to repairing the diseased valves. Repair of aortic and mitral valves is mainly possible if there is regurgitation pathology without significant calcification and/or destruction of the valve apparatus. Sir

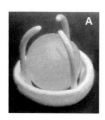 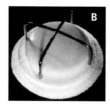 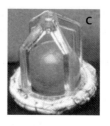 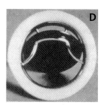

(A–D) Older mechanical prostheses:

> High profile-poor haemodynamics and larger gradients across the valves
> Less durable (more stress fractures)
> More thrombogenic
> Need anticoagulation
> No resistance against infection
> Noisy

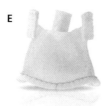 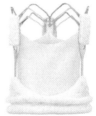

(E,F) Newer tissue valves (3F). Sutureless implant comes with self-expanding Nitinol frame:

> Low profile-optimal haemodynamics and low gradients for the given size
> Durable as they mimic native valve
> Minimal thrombogenicity
> No need of anticoagulation
> Less prone to calcification, degradation and infection
> Silent
> Handle well and easy to implant

Fig. 1 Comparison between old and new valve prostheses (photographs reproduced with permission from ATS Medical Inc.).

Magdi Yacoub in the UK and Dr T. David in Canada have done pioneering work in aortic valve preservation techniques. Mitral valve repair surgery is credited to Dr A. Carpentier who systematically analysed different pathologies of the mitral valve and laid down their classification method. He pioneered various ways of repairing the mitral valve that has helped to lower the mortality of mitral valve surgery from around 5% to 1–2%. Additional benefits of repairing the valve rather than replacing it lie in the fact that there is no need for anticoagulation. The incidence of thrombo-embolism and haemolysis can be minimised and, most importantly, the morphology of left ventricle and mitral valve is maintained, thereby preserving left ventricle function.

Key point 3

- Type of prosthesis, repair techniques and the less invasive access to the valve are the three directions of the current cardiac valvular research.

In the near future, we shall be able to cultivate tailor-made valves in the laboratory for an individual from his or her own cell culture, ready for implantation. Many investigators have already done work in this area[7] and stem cell research has played a pivotal role.

PERFUSION TECHNOLOGY

Over the last few years, all components of perfusion technology have changed dramatically. Fifty years ago, large rotating drums and the discs that were used for oxygenators occupied almost one room in the operating theatre. Modern membrane oxygenators can fit in the palm of the hand and are as efficient as natural lungs in oxygenating the blood. Newer centrifugal pumps are small and disposable. They minimise the chances of air embolism and haemolysis. They also increase safety by being afterload dependent. Pulsatile pumps can provide pulsatile flow thus mimicking natural flow patterns. Tubing is made from durable polymer thus minimising the chances of embolism by shear forces. Tubing is available with heparin coating, thus minimising systemic effects of heparin and protamin. Filters, alarms and other monitoring gauges that are integrated, make perfusion very safe.

Percutaneous catheter technology has also been extensively developed, making it possible to establish cardiopulmonary bypass, without making any incisions (Heartport), thus helping in robotic surgery. Percutaneous insertion of catheters can also be used for deploying ventricular assist devices (VADs) in failing hearts. As the experience with cardiopulmonary bypass technology grew, its role became diverse. Cardiopulmonary bypass can be used for treatment of hypothermia, near–drowning, certain drug toxicities (tricyclic antidepressants) and pulmonary embolism. It can also be used in treating certain malignancies such as malignant melanoma, renal cell carcinoma involving IVC and large neurovascular tumours. Perfusion technology is being advanced in the fields of spinal protection (left heart bypass) and cerebral protection (antegrade or retrograde cerebral perfusion) during trauma and major aortic arch surgery.

Key point 4

- Perfusion has become safer, its components miniaturised and its uses diversified.

OFF-PUMP SURGERY

Since the late 1950s, cardiopulmonary bypass has been in use in the practice of cardiac surgery. Although it has proved to be a safe and useful tool in supporting the circulation of the body whilst the heart and lungs are not working during cardiac surgery, cardiopulmonary bypass cannot be employed without its untoward side effects on different organ systems. Prolonged cardiopulmonary bypass is known to give rise to renal dysfunction, neurocognitive changes, ARDS, coagulation abnormalities and gastrointestinal dysfunction in the forms of pancreatitis and gut ischaemia.

Table 1 Terminologies used in context of off-pump surgery

OPCAB	Off-pump coronary artery bypass (usually via sternotomy)
MIDCAB	Minimally invasive direct coronary artery bypass (usually via small anterior thoracotomy)
Endo ACAB	Endoscopically assisted coronary artery bypass (IMA is harvested endoscopically and anastomosis is performed via a small incision)
TECAB	Totally endoscopic coronary artery bypass (IMA harvesting and anastomosis endoscopically through small ports)
PADCAB	Perfusion-assisted direct coronary artery bypass (perfusion is maintained distal to coronary anastomosis with the use of special catheters)
Aesop, Zeus, Da Vinci	Robotic arms being developed for the use of harvesting and anastomosis
VATS	Video-assisted thoracoscopic surgery (port access, endoscopic)

In order to minimise these effects, many surgeons turned their attention to cardiac surgery without the use of cardiopulmonary bypass, through minimal access (as against standard midsternotomy) or both. The last 10 years or so have seen an evolution of cardiac surgery in these fields. In this context, various terminologies have emerged that are explained in Table 1.

OPCAB minimises many of the untoward effects of cardiopulmonary bypass on the renal system.[8] Avoidance of cardiopulmonary bypass may help preservation of glomerular and tubular function and minimise renal damage.[9] OPCABs also reduce transfusion rates, incidence of atrial fibrillation and risks of neurocognitive dysfunction. Its major benefits may be seen in patients with multiple co-morbidities such as CRF, poor LV and PVD.[10] Reduction in neurocognitive dysfunction is seen maximally in cases where surgery is performed with a no-touch technique to aorta (total arterial revascularisation with use of Y-grafts or jump grafts). This benefit is offset if multiple side biting clamps are applied to the aorta for proximal anastomoses of the venous grafts.

MIDCAB can be performed either unilaterally or bilaterally. Complete revascularisation of the myocardium is only possible with this technique if one or two coronaries are diseased. If multiple coronaries are diseased, the one of maximal prognostic or symptomatic significance is bypassed with MIDCAB, and then the cardiologist can stent the remaining vessels at a later date. This technique of revascularisation is called hybrid revascularisation. Although large incisions and cardiopulmonary bypass can be avoided with this method, its long-term benefits are still unproven.

With VATS or port access surgery, large incisions can be avoided. This improves cosmesis, and minimises bleeding, pain and hospital stay. Video-assisted surgery is currently extensively used in various subspecialities of surgery; however, its role in cardiac surgery is still in its infancy. The following procedures can be performed with this technique: (i) device manipulation; (ii) division of left SVC or any other collateral vessel; (iii) relief of LVOT obstruction; (iv) LV thrombectomy; (v) epicardial pacing lead insertion; and (vi) muscular VSD repair.

ROBOTIC SURGERY

Robotic surgery is a new frontier in the field of cardiac surgery. It can be performed with or without the use of cardiopulmonary bypass. Early generations of robots used software that recognised the surgeon's voice command or head movements, and implemented the required task with the robotic arm. Newer robots have evolved and are capable of performing more complex tasks. The robotic arms also have multiple degrees of freedom mimicking a human arm and are able to perform fine anastomoses whilst the surgeon is sitting remote from the patient and is giving commands on a console with a joy stick.

Currently the following operations are performed with the help of a robot: coronary artery bypass surgery; MV repair; ASD closure; AF ablation; pericardiectomy / pericardial window; and closure of PDA.

The potential advantages and disadvantages of robotic technology are summarised in Table 2.

Table 2 Advantages and disadvantages of robotic surgery

Advantages	Disadvantages
Better dexterity, no tremors	Lack of tactile feedback
Less fatigue to surgeons (better mental and physical ergonomics)	Time-consuming preparation and the procedure
Small incision-less pain, less bleeding, better cosmesis	Steep and tall learning curve
Reduced stay in hospital	Expensive to install
	Lack of adequate evidence base for routine procedure like CABG

Key point 5

- Cardiac surgery can be safely performed without cardiopulmonary bypass and with or without the use of robot.

MANAGEMENT OF HEART FAILURE

The number of patients with failing hearts is on the increase in the developed world. Drugs like β-blockers, ACE inhibitors, spironolactone and digoxin have all contributed to lowering the mortality due to heart failure. They also increase event–free survival and reduce hospital admission in patients with heart failure. Statins and other cholesterol-lowering drugs play a pivotal role in primary and secondary prophylaxis of coronary atherosclerosis, thus helping to reduce the number of heart failure patients.

In ischaemic cardiomyopathy, as scar tissue replaces the conduction pathway, there is de-synchronised contraction of the ventricular myocardium. This leads to wastage of energy and decreased efficiency of the myocardial pump. Cardiac resynchronisation therapy enables synchronised contractions of the ventricles by simultaneous biventricular pacing, thus improving cardiac contractility.[11]

The surgical options for treatment of heart failure have also widened in the last decade. Revascularising ischaemic myocardium by CABG and rectifying leaking mitral valve with repair or replacement significantly improves the symptoms of breathlessness and angina and the prognosis of these patients.

Cardiomyoplasty and partial left ventricle resection (Batista procedure) were performed initially, but have fallen out of use due to lack of evidence of their benefits and the high mortality associated with such procedures.

Endoventricular circular patch plasty (Dor procedure) restores left ventricle geometry and gets rid of non-functional aneurysmal areas of the left ventricle. Early results with this procedure are promising in heart failure management. External ventricular constraint devices such as the Acorn device, Myosplint and Heart Booster have shown a reduction in ventricular dilatation and their wall stresses, thus improving ejection fraction.[12,13] LVADs and total artificial hearts are used either as destination therapy in heart failure patients or as a bridge to recovery or bridge to transplant. There usually is marked haemodynamic and phenotypic profile improvement with these devices. In the REMATCH trial there was 48% reduction in the risk of death in LVAD cohort.[14]

Key point 6

- Better understanding of aetiopathologies and the mechanisms of heart failure has given rise to various medical and surgical treatments with improved results.

FUTURE ADVANCES

There is no doubt that technology will play an immense role in the future of cardiac surgery. Robots will be more sophisticated and complex and will have the potential of performing surgery without the help of humans! Valves will be cultured in laboratories and hearts will be cloned. We will be in a position whereby blood substitutes will be used, thus preserving the patient's own blood for later use. Stem cell research will hold the key to many future developments in the field of medicine.

Key points for clinical practice

- Newer diagnostic modalities have led to early detection and better management of cardiac pathologies.

- Development of anaesthesia, blood bank and critical care management has helped achieve better results of cardiac surgery.

- Type of prosthesis, repair techniques and the less invasive access to the valve are the three directions of the current cardiac valvular research.

Key points for clinical practice *(continued)*

- Perfusion has become safer, its components miniaturised and its uses diversified.

- Cardiac surgery can be safely performed without cardiopulmonary bypass and with or without the use of robot.

- Better understanding of aetiopathologies and the mechanisms of heart failure has given rise to various medical and surgical treatments with improved results.

References

1. Gan TJ, Arrowsmith JE. The oesophageal Doppler monitor: a safe means of monitoring the circulation. *BMJ* 1997; **315**: 893–894.
2. Jonas M, Tanser S. Lithium dilution measurement of cardiac output and arterial pulse waveform analysis: an indicator dilution calibrated beat-by-beat system for continuous estimation of cardiac output. *Curr Opin Crit Care* 2002; **8**: 257–261.
3. Binder T, Globits S, Zangeneh M *et al*. Three-dimensional echocardiography using a transoesophageal imaging probe. Potentials and technical considerations. *Eur Heart J* 1996; **17**: 487–489.
4. Mohammed Abd El-Rahman S, Khatri G, Nanda N *et al*. Transesophageal three-dimensional echocardiographic assessment of normal and stenosed coronary arteries. *Echocardiography* 1996; **13**: 503–510.
5. Binder T. Three-dimensional echocardiography – principles and promises. *J Clin Basic Cardiol* 2002; **5**: 149–152.
6. Nashef SA, Roques F, Michel P, Gauducheau E, Lemeshow S, Salamon R. European system for cardiac operative risk evaluation (EuroSCORE). *Eur J Cardiothorac Surg* 1999; **16**: 9–13.
7. Gabbieri D, Dohmen PM, Linneweber J, Lembcke A, Braun JP, Konertz W. Ross procedure with tissue-engineered heart valve in complex congenital aortic valve disease. *J Thorac Cardiovasc Surg* 2007; **133**: 1088–1089.
8. Stallwood MI, Grayson AD, Mills K, Scawn ND. Acute renal failure in coronary artery bypass surgery: independent effect of cardiopulmonary bypass. *Ann Thorac Surg* 2004; **77**: 968–972.
9. Ascione R, Nason G, Al-Ruzzeh S, Ko C, Ciulli F, Angelini GD. Coronary revascularisation with or without cardiopulmonary bypass in patients with preoperative nondialysis-dependent renal insufficiency. *Ann Thorac Surg* 2001; **72**: 2020–2025.
10. Mack MJ. Beating heart surgery: does it make a difference? *Am Heart Hosp J* 2003; **1**: 149–157.
11. Hare JM. Cardiac-resynchronization therapy for heart failure. *N Engl J Med* 2002; **346**: 1902–1905.
12. McCarthy PM, Takagaki M, Ochiai Y *et al*. Device-based change in left ventricular shape: a new concept for the treatment of dilated cardiomyopathy. *J Thorac Cardiovasc Surg* 2001; **122**: 482–490.
13. Konertz WF, Shapland JE, Hotz H *et al*. Passive containment and reverse remodelling by a novel textile cardiac support device. *Circulation* 2001; **104 (Suppl 1)**: 1270–1275.
14. Rose EA, Gelijns AC, Moskowitz AJ *et al*. Long-term use of LV assist device for end stage heart failure. *N Engl J Med* 2001; **345**: 1435–1443.

Michael Lewis Jonathan Hyde
Christopher Munsch

7

Penetrating cardiac injury

There has recently been an increase in penetrating trauma in the UK.[1] Penetrating cardiac injury is a major contributor to mortality and is immediately lethal in up to 60% of cases. However, some patients arrive at hospital alive or suitable for resuscitation.[2,3]

Approximately 15% of penetrating cardiac injury deaths have evidence of cardiac tamponade.[4] Around 80–90% of patients with thoracic stab wounds present with signs of tamponade.[5] This is a reversible potential cause of death and correct management is associated with improved survival following penetrating cardiac injury.[6,7] There is, therefore, a group of patients in whom prompt surgical intervention might lead to improved outcome and survival.[8,9]

In most cases of non-fatal penetrating cardiac injury, emergency surgery is needed immediately. This will, therefore, not usually allow cardiothoracic surgical input. The Definitive Surgical Trauma Skills (DSTS) Course (convened jointly by The Royal College of Surgeons of England, the Royal Defence Medical College and the Uniformed Services University of the Health Sciences in the USA) addresses this by delivering a practical programme of surgical trauma care, and includes a section on chest trauma management. The DSTS course provides the basis for the text of this chapter and assumes that ATLS principles have already been followed.[10]

Michael Lewis BSc MD FRCS(CTh)
Consultant Cardiothoracic Surgeon, Sussex Cardiac Centre, Royal Sussex County Hospital, Brighton BN2 5BE, UK

Jonathan Hyde BSc MD FRCS(CTh)
Consultant Cardiothoracic Surgeon, Sussex Cardiac Centre, Royal Sussex County Hospital, Brighton BN2 5BE, UK

Christopher Munsch ChM FRCS(CTh) (for correspondence)
Consultant Cardiothoracic Surgeon, Leeds General Infirmary, Great George Street, Leeds LS1 3EX, UK. E-mail: chris.munsch@tiscali.co.uk

Key points 1–4

- Penetrating cardiac injuries are fatal in a high percentage of cases.

- Most penetrating cardiac injuries need to be dealt with by non-cardiothoracic surgeons at time of presentation.

- Application of straightforward techniques can control a significant proportion of penetrating cardiac injuries that reach hospital.

- Appropriate, timely intervention can save lives.

AETIOLOGY

Penetrating cardiac injury may occur as a result of: (i) stab wounds; (ii) ballistic wounds, including gunshot and missile injuries; or (iii) impalement. In the UK, penetrating cardiac injury most commonly results from stab wounds, usually caused by knives. Gunshot wounds to the heart are rare (but increasing in frequency) and are significantly more lethal than stab wounds, with only 11% of victims arriving at hospital alive (40% following stabbing).[11,12] Gunshot wounds transfer large amounts of energy to the body due to the kinetic energy released into the surrounding tissues as the bullet passes through the body.

Missile injuries can be high or low velocity, and one should be aware these devices often cause thermal/blast injuries, with other mechanisms of tissue damage.

Impalement injury can present specific difficulties as there are frequently problems moving the patient.

Key points 5 and 6

- Stabbing is the commonest cause of penetrating cardiac injury in the UK.

- Gunshot injuries are increasing in incidence.

MANAGEMENT

DECISION MAKING

Patients with penetrating cardiac injury secondary to stabbing often have an entry wound over the praecordium or the left chest, but remote entry wounds are well described.[13] Assessment of surface wounds is unreliable, the history of injury being more important. Where the knife is still *in situ*, removal must only be undertaken in the operating theatre. If the patient is stable, consideration should be given to transfer to a specialist unit first.

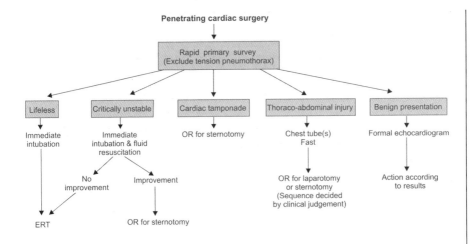

Fig.1 An algorithm for management modified from Degiannis *et al.*[7]

Penetrating cardiac injury will not always occur in isolation and injury to surrounding structures should always be considered. More stable patients may be able to undergo further pre-operative investigations, such as echocardiography or computed tomography (CT). One series showed two-dimensional echocardiography to be 90% sensitive and 97% specific for the diagnosis of cardiac penetration in stable penetrating cardiac injury.[14] Pericardiocentesis is unreliable.[15]

Triage is fundamental to the assessment of penetrating cardiac injury as many patients are unsalvageable.[16] Patients who have had no signs of life (unconscious patients with no clinically detectable signs of life; electrocardiography may show the presence of occasional QRS complexes or may be grossly abnormal) for 5 min (no endotracheal intubation) or 10 min (intubated) are unlikely to respond to resuscitative thoracotomy.[17] Outcome is also significantly worse for patients who have their surgery outside the operating theatre. In some situations, such as a witnessed arrest, an emergency department thoracotomy is appropriate. An algorithm for management is given in Degiannis *et al.*[7] (Fig.1).

Confirmed penetrating cardiac injury mandates surgical exploration. Successful emergency department thoracotomy is only a temporary and life-saving measure to facilitate a later, definitive procedure in the operating theatre, and should only be performed if there is no alternative.

Thoraco-abdominal injuries are problematic as thoracotomy and laparotomy are often both needed – but in which order? Focused Abdominal Sonogram for Trauma (FAST) scans can aid the decision, and are increasingly available.

DEFINITIVE MANAGEMENT

DSTS teaches various methods of access for thoracic trauma, including left anterior thoracotomy, bilateral anterior thoracotomy and median sternotomy. The choice of incision and their limitations must be considered (Table 1). DSTS recommends left anterior thoracotomy or bilateral anterior thoracotomy as

Table 1 Methods of access for thoracic trauma, choices and limitations

	Left anterior thoracotomy	Bilateral anterior thoracotomy	Median sternotomy
Rapidity and ease of incision	***	**	*
Specialised equipment requirement	*	**	***
Access to vital structures	*	***	***
Ease of closure	**	*	**

first-line access, due to minimal equipment requirements and excellent, rapid exposure.

• Left anterior thoracotomy allows immediate relief of tamponade and internal cardiac massage. Its disadvantage is that little else can be achieved as only a very small area of the heart can be visualised. If the laceration is not immediately visible, then extension into a bilateral anterior thoracotomy is mandated.

• Bilateral anterior thoracotomy allows quick access to, and excellent visualisation of, all three thoracic cavities (left and right pleurae and pericardium).

• Median sternotomy may occasionally be the most appropriate incision, but requires sternal division; if performed incorrectly, it can be difficult to close.

Peri-operative care

• Do not forget antibiotics and anti-tetanus

• Many penetrating injuries introduce foreign material into the wound track; debride these as necessary

• Prevent or treat hypothermia, which is common in trauma and exacerbated by thoracotomy. Hypothermia affects physiological processes such as coagulation and tissue perfusion.

Preparation

• Inform the patient (if conscious) and the entire team what to expect

• Contact the cardiothoracic surgeons

• Rapidly position, prepare and drape the patient, whilst maintaining cardiopulmonary resuscitation

• Double-lumen intubation is unnecessary and time-wasting.

Incisions – left anterior thoracotomy

• 4th or 5th ICS from mid-axillary line to sternal edge

- Incise through skin/fat/muscle onto the upper surface of the rib
- Incise intercostal muscles and open pleura digitally with a finger sweep
- Insert retractor and open wide (disregard rib fractures)
- Open the pericardium longitudinally 2 cm anterior to the phrenic nerve
- Relieve tamponade and commence internal massage if necessary
- If bleeding source is obvious, digitally occlude it, and expedite fluid resuscitation
- If bleeding continues and source not obvious, immediately convert to bilateral anterior thoracotomy.

Incisions – bilateral anterior thoracotomy

- Duplicate the left anterior thoracotomy incision on the right
- Divide the sternum/midline tissue transversely with heavy scissors to join the incisions
- Insert a retractor and open widely.

Incisions – median sternotomy

- Incise through skin/fat/muscle to the sternal periosteum, from jugular notch to xiphoid process
- Identify the mid-line and divide the sternum using a saw
- Place a retractor between the sternal edges and open widely
- Divide/sweep away the mediastinal fat to identify the pericardial sac
- Be aware that the innominate vein lies in the fat superiorly
- Incise the pericardial sac longitudinally, releasing the tamponade.

Intrapericardial procedures

If the chest is opened by median sternotomy or bilateral anterior thoracotomy, the thymus, if present, should be divided, taking care not to damage the innominate vein.

Open the pericardium as described above. The left and right phrenic nerves lie in a lateral position on the pericardium running in a craniocaudal direction anterior to the right and left hilae. Great care should be taken to preserve these nerves as damage will lead to diaphragmatic paralysis and severe respiratory compromise.

Caution should be shown if the heart is beating normally as handling the heart can cause arrhythmias and haemodynamic compromise. Whilst establishing a life-sustaining cardiac rhythm, the bleeding point(s) should be identified and digital control obtained. This may necessitate a brief discontinuation of ventilation to allow an improved view of the intrapericardial contents.

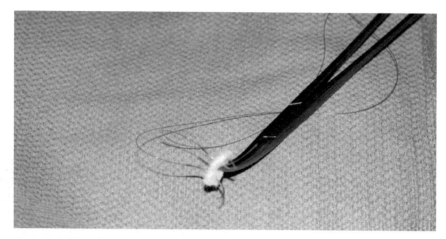

Fig. 2 A Teflon pledget. The double-armed suture is first passed through the pledget and then through the tissue. A second pledget is the mounted and the suture tied.

Once the bleeding is controlled digitally, one can further resuscitate the patient and plan definitive repair of the cardiac wound(s).

Opening of the right and left pleurae should be undertaken (at an appropriate stage) to inspect for extrapericardial injuries.

Suture choice

Most cardiac repairs can be achieved using a 5-0 or 4-0 polypropylene suture. A useful size is a 25-mm round-bodied needle. This facilitates the passage of the suture into the beating heart, allowing full-thickness bites and recovery of the needle in one pass. The benefit of a needle of this size is that, if digital control is being applied, it can be passed through the wound beneath the occluding finger without need to remove the pressure.

The use of pledgets (either proprietary Teflon or cut from the patient's pericardium; Fig 2) is necessary if the tissues will not hold sutures well or the defect is in a high-pressure chamber such as the ventricle. The pledgets spread

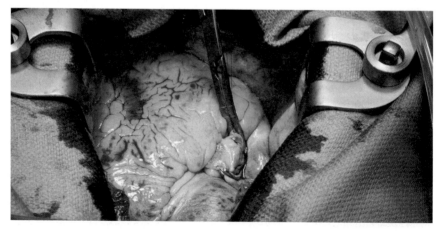

Fig. 3 A side-biting clamp used to control bleeding from the right atrial appendage.

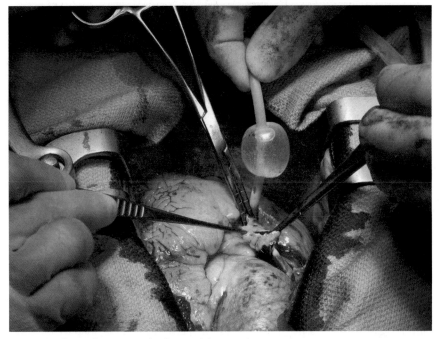

Fig. 4 A Foley catheter can also be used (see text).

the load of the suture and prevent the stitch from 'cheese-wiring' through the tissue.

Repair techniques

The location of the cardiac injury dictates the technique that can be used to repair the injury. Some atrial and aortic injuries can be controlled with the application of a vascular side-biting clamp. The damaged area can then be

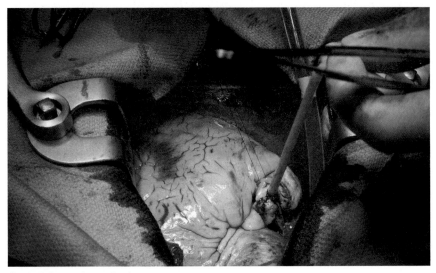

Fig. 5 Foley catheter *in situ*.

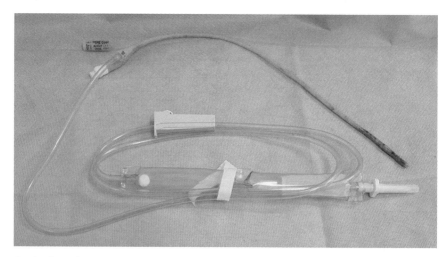

Fig. 6 The Foley catheter can be connected to an infusion set to allow rapid transfusion.

over-sewn and the clamp removed once control is achieved (Fig. 3). Be careful not to retract on the clamp too forcefully as the atria are fragile and can tear easily.

Another useful technique to control bleeding is with the use of a Foley catheter (Figs 4 and 5). The tip of the catheter is inserted directly through the injury and the balloon inflated with saline. Gentle counter-traction will seal the hole and allow the surrounding area to be visualised. A clamp must be placed proximally across the lumen of the catheter to prevent back-bleeding. Sutures can then be placed in a purse-string fashion to control the defect. It is worthwhile having spare Foley catheters as the balloon may be punctured by the needle whilst placing these sutures. This technique is usually used for atrial or ventricular injuries due to their large cavity size.

A further advantage of this technique is that it can be used as a central line (Fig. 6) to restore volume rapidly. A fluid infusion 'giving-set' can be connected directly to the catheter so that blood and fluids can be given directly into the heart.

Coronary artery injuries

These injuries are difficult to manage. Injury close to (but not involving) a coronary artery can be managed by running a horizontal mattress suture under the epicardial vessel. Pledgeted sutures are particularly useful in this situation as they help to form a 'bridge' on which the coronary artery can lie.

Bleeding from small coronary arteries can be controlled by ligation of the injured vessel, with only limited (and non-fatal) areas of infarction. Using this technique on proximal major vessels, however, is associated with a 40% mortality.[18]

If available, coronary shunts as utilised in 'off-pump' coronary surgery may be used to control bleeding while arrangements are made for transfer to a cardiothoracic surgery centre for definitive treatment.[19]

Posterior cardiac injuries

The natural sequence of management is such that anterior wounds tend to be dealt with first, as they are usually the most easily seen. However, the posterior surface of the heart should be carefully inspected to check for damage (commonly seen with 'through-and-through' injuries).

Lifting the heart can cause circulatory embarrassment as the venous return to the heart is impeded by such manoeuvres. This part of the operation should, therefore, be conducted in close discussion with the anaesthetist who should monitor the patient's circulatory status. Restoring the heart back into its anatomical position in the pericardial well will allow the circulation to recover in most instances.

It may, therefore, be necessary to approach posterior injuries in a step-wise fashion allowing the heart to recover between the operative steps of placing and tying the suture.

CLOSURE

Once the cardiac injury has been repaired, a thorough check for haemostasis should be made. Any thoracic cavity that has been opened needs draining. Place an apical and basal drain in each pleural cavity. Apical drains are placed anteriorly and basal drains are placed posteriorly (AAA for anterior/apical/air, and BBB for back/basal/blood). The drains should be of a good calibre to prevent blockage (28–32-G) and should all be connected to underwater-seal bottles.

Closure – left anterior thoracotomy

It is not common to close a left anterior thoracotomy incision in isolation unless the diagnosis is wrong and no tamponade has been found. In most cases, either the incision is converted to a bilateral anterior thoracotomy (see below) or the patient, once stabilised, is transferred to the operating theatre for a definitive procedure. Once there, the closure follows the principles outlined for bilateral anterior thoracotomy below.

Closure – bilateral anterior thoracotomy (clamshell)

Once satisfactory intrathoracic haemostasis has been achieved (ensure the mammary arteries are not bleeding prior to closure) and appropriate intercostal and mediastinal drains have been inserted, the chest can be closed.

Closure is commenced by re-approximating the ribs with three or four 'figure-of-eight' sutures using a heavy absorbable suture (*e.g.* 0-vicryl), on each side. Once all the sutures are placed, they can be tied. The anterior ribs naturally lie further apart than the posterior ones, therefore the anterior ribs are stabilised with the sutures rather than closely approximated.

Make a final check of haemostasis and the position of the drains to ensure that they sit appropriately within the chest and are connected to the underwater seal circuits.

Sternal approximation is performed with either a similar heavy suture or a stainless steel wire (see below). The muscle layer should be closed with a 2-0 absorbable suture. Close the fat layer and skin in the routine manner.

Closure – median sternotomy

The sternal edges are checked for bleeding and once dry (marrow always oozes) the sternal wires are placed. The wires are 5-gauge stainless steel sutures.

Place three wires in the manubrium and at least four in the remaining body of the sternum. Place the drains on low pressure (5–10 cmH$_2$O) suction. Pull the sternal edges together by crossing the wires and twist until secure. Cut the wires and flatten the stumps onto the sternum so that they will not protrude through the skin postoperatively.

Use a non-absorbable suture to close the linea alba. Close the fat layer and skin in the routine manner.

Key points 7–9

- Emergency thoracotomy should be directed at relief of tamponade and attaining haemodynamic stability, followed by definitive haemorrhage control.

- The choice of incision is crucial. Advantages and limitations of each should be considered as part of the resuscitation process.

- Emergency thoracotomy should be performed in the operating theatre unless there is no alternative.

POSTOPERATIVE MANAGEMENT

All patients with significant chest trauma, particularly penetrating cardiac injury, will require intensive care unit management to monitor the patient appropriately and optimise physiological parameters. Depending on the degree of wound contamination, prophylactic postoperative antibiotics may be required. Once the patient is ready to be weaned from the ventilator, analgesia requirements should be considered carefully. Patients who have undergone a clamshell incision may require either a thoracic epidural infusion or patient-controlled analgesia to obtain adequate pain relief to allow the individual to cough and perform physiotherapy adequately.

Postoperatively, all patients should have a chest radiograph to check the position of intravenous lines and chest tubes and to rule out any significant residual pneumothoraces or fluid collections.

Penetrating cardiac injuries may rarely traverse the cardiac septum or affect the intracardiac valves.[20-22] Unless the damage is severe, these injuries can often be managed conservatively, particularly in the acute stage. They should be followed up with routine echocardiograms to guide the necessity and timing of definitive repair. Such defects should be discussed with a cardiothoracic surgical unit.

Key points for clinical practice

- Penetrating cardiac injuries are fatal in a high percentage of cases.

- Most penetrating cardiac injuries need to be dealt with by non-cardiothoracic surgeons at time of presentation.

- Application of straightforward techniques can control a significant proportion of penetrating cardiac injuries that reach hospital.

- Appropriate, timely intervention can save lives.

- Stabbing is the commonest cause of penetrating cardiac injury in the UK.

- Gunshot injuries are increasing in incidence.

- Emergency thoracotomy should be directed at relief of tamponade and attaining haemodynamic stability, followed by definitive haemorrhage control.

- The choice of incision is crucial. Advantages and limitations of each should be considered as part of the resuscitation process.

- Emergency thoracotomy should be performed in the operating theatre unless there is no alternative.

References

1. BBC. 2008 <http://news.bbc.co.uk/1/hi/uk/7510901.stm>.
2. Campbell NC, Thomson SR, Muckart DJ, Meumann CM, Van Middelkoop I, Botha JB. Review of 1198 cases of penetrating cardiac trauma. *Br J Surg* 1997; **84**: 1737–1740.
3. von Oppell UO, Bautz P, De Groot M. Penetrating thoracic injuries: what we have learnt. *Thorac Cardiovasc Surg* 2000; **48**: 55–61.
4. Okada Y, Suzuki H, Mukaida M, Ishiyama I. Penetrating cardiac injuries. A pathological analysis of 20 autopsy cases. *Am J Forensic Med Pathol* 1990; **11**: 144–148.
5. Ivatury R. Rohman M. In: Turney SZ, Rodriquez A, Cowley R. (eds) *Management of Cardiothoracic Trauma*. Baltimore, MD: Williams and Wilkins, 1990; 311–347.
6. Kavolius J, Golocovsky M, Champion HR. Predictors of outcome in patients who have sustained trauma and who undergo emergency thoracotomy. *Arch Surg* 1993; **128**: 1158–1162.
7. Degiannis E, Loogna P, Doll D, Bonanno F, Bowley DM, Smith MD. Penetrating cardiac injuries: Recent experience in South Africa. *World J Surg* 2006; **30**: 1258–1264.
8. Working Group, Ad Hoc Subcommittee on Outcomes, American College of Surgeons Committee on Trauma. Practice management guidelines for emergency department thoracotomy. *J Am Coll Surg* 2001; **193**: 303–309.
9. Arreola-Risa C, Rhee P, Boyle EM, Maier RV, Jurkovich GG, Foy HM. Factors influencing outcome in stab wounds of the heart. *Am J Surg* 1995; **169**: 553–556.
10. American College of Surgeons. *Advanced Trauma Life Support*, 7th edn. Chicago, IL: American College of Surgeons, 2004.
11. Meredith J, Trunkey D. Thoracic gunshot wounds. In: Ordog G. (ed) *Management of Gunshot Wounds*. New York: Elsevier, 1988.
12. Karrel R, Shaffer MA, Franaszek JB. Emergency diagnosis, resuscitation, and treatment of acute penetrating cardiac trauma. *Ann Emerg Med* 1982; **11**: 504–517.

13. Demetriades D, Rabinowitz B, Sofianos C. Emergency room thoracotomy for stab wounds to the chest and neck. J Trauma 1987; **27**: 483–485.
14. Jimenez E, Martin M, Krukenkamp I, Barrett J. Subxiphoid pericardiotomy versus echocardiography: a prospective evaluation of the diagnosis of occult penetrating cardiac injury. *Surgery* 1990; **108**: 676–680.
15. Arom KV, Richardson JD, Webb G, Grover FL, Trinkle JK. Subxiphoid pericardial window in patients with suspected traumatic pericardial tamponade. *Ann Thorac Surg* 1977; **23**: 545–549.
16. Tyburski JG, Astra L, Wilson RF, Dente C, Steffes C. Factors affecting prognosis with penetrating wounds of the heart. *J Trauma* 2000; **48**: 587–591.
17. Velmahos GC, Degiannis E, Souter I, Allwood AC, Saadia R. Outcome of a strict policy on emergency department thoracotomies. *Arch Surg* 1995; **130**: 774–777.
18. Rea WJ, Sugg WL, Wilson LC, Webb WR, Ecker RR. Coronary artery lacerations; an analysis of 22 patients. *Ann Thorac Surg* 1969; **7**: 518–528.
19. Fedalen PA, Bard MR, Piacentino 3rd V *et al*. Intraluminal shunt placement and off-pump coronary revascularization for coronary artery stab wound. *J Trauma* 2001; **50**: 133–135.
20. Richardson JE, Duncan WJ, Bharadwaj B, McMeekin JD. Traumatic wound of the heart: value of intraoperative colour Doppler flow imaging. *Can J Cardiol* 1988; **4**: 338–340.
21. Goldman AP, Kotler MN, Goldberg SE, Parameswaran R, Parry W. The uses of two-dimensional Doppler echocardiographic techniques preoperatively and postoperatively in a ventricular septal defect caused by penetrating trauma. *Ann Thorac Surg* 1985; **40**: 625–627.
22. Asfaw I, Thoms NW, Arbulu A. Interventricular septal defects from penetrating injuries of the heart: a report of 12 cases and review of the literature. *J Thorac Cardiovasc Surg* 1975; **69**: 450–457.

Jan Jansen Malcolm A. Loudon

8

Investigation and management of blunt abdominal trauma

Trauma remains the fourth leading cause of death in Western societies, and the leading cause of death in the first four decades of life.[1] The predominant mechanism in the UK is blunt injury. Precise data on injury patterns are lacking, but valuable information can be extracted from the recent NCEPOD report on the provision of trauma care in England and Wales. Nearly three-quarters of patients had been involved in a road traffic collision or a fall from height, mechanisms generally associated with a blunt mode of injury.[1] Almost one-fifth of patients had abdominal injuries.[1] Blunt abdominal trauma, therefore, constitutes a considerable workload.

Intra-abdominal haemorrhage remains one of the commonest causes of death after trauma,[2] and missed abdominal injuries are a frequent cause of morbidity and late mortality. The quality of trauma management may thus contribute to avoidable morbidity and the attendant social and financial costs.

In the UK, it has been suggested that almost 60% of trauma patients receive a standard of care considered to be suboptimal.[1]

The aim of this chapter is to provide an overview of the investigation and management of adult patients with blunt abdominal trauma.

MECHANISMS OF INJURY

Blunt abdominal trauma may result in injury to intra-abdominal organs by two discrete mechanisms – direct compression and deceleration resulting in shearing forces. Compression may result from a direct blow or from a

Jan Jansen FRCS (for correspondence)
Consultant Surgeon, Department of Surgery, Aberdeen Royal Infirmary, Aberdeen AB25 2ZN, UK.
E-mail: jan.jansen@nhs.net

Malcolm A. Loudon MD FRCSEd(Gen)
Consultant Surgeon, Department of Surgery, Aberdeen Royal Infirmary, Aberdeen AB25 2ZN, UK.
E-mail: malcolml@doctors.org.uk

concussive force causing the casualty to be propelled against, or restrained by, another object. Compressive forces most commonly result in solid visceral injury to spleen, liver and kidneys and discrete symptoms and signs should raise a high index of suspicion for such injuries particularly if the history is consistent with an appropriate mechanism, such as a single blow to the left or right upper quadrant. In this context, the mechanism of injury is that of crushing or tearing resulting in subcapsular haemorrhage or parenchymal disruption.

Less commonly, the hollow viscera may be injured as a result of compression, particularly if the abdomen is restrained or compressed by a fixed object such as a seat belt. The mechanism of injury is a transient rise in intraluminal pressure sufficient to cause visceral rupture. One example may be seen when a particularly sinister combination of injuries occurs as a result of pancreaticoduodenal compression against the lumbar spine.

Key point 1

- Blunt intra-abdominal injury results from direct compression or deceleration.

Deceleration results in tearing at points of fixity. This can result in solid organ injuries such as hepatic tears along the ligamentum teres or shearing into the splenic pedicle. The relative length and mobility of the mesentery at its attachment and its fixity at the point of origin may result in haemorrhage from torn mesenteric vessels or ischaemia due to intimal thrombosis.

INDICATORS OF RISK

Attention should be paid to surrogate markers of risk in assessing the trauma patient. Death of a casualty at scene, ejection, intrusion into the passenger compartment or extraction of one or more casualties from a vehicle have all been identified as strong predictors of a high risk of intra-abdominal injury following motor vehicle accidents. Falls from a height of more than 4 m are also highly predictive of significant injury.

INJURY PATTERNS

Certain patterns or constellations of injury are well recognised but remain pitfalls for the unwary or inexperienced. A good example is the lap seat belt wearer who experiences a forced flexion injury. A seat belt bruise may be evident and appropriate imaging reveals a lumbar spine fracture. An abdominal computed tomography (CT) scan is the imaging modality of choice in the haemodynamically stable patient and careful consideration should be given to the risks and benefits of using oral contrast as subtle signs, particularly in relation to pancreaticoduodenal injuries, may be missed.

Injuries outwith the abdomen are also important indicators of an increased risk of intra-abdominal injury. Injury above and below the diaphragm, markers of high energy transfer such as proximal rib fractures or major pelvic fracture dislocations are some examples.

INVESTIGATING BLUNT ABDOMINAL TRAUMA

The presentation of blunt abdominal trauma ranges from the dramatic (such as a patient involved in a road traffic collision or explosion, presenting with profound haemodynamic instability due to major haemorrhage) to the subtle, early signs of an otherwise well patient with a hollow viscus injury following relatively trivial and localised trauma. Both investigative and management strategies must take into account these widely different presentations, and their differing clinical priorities.

Diagnosing intra-abdominal injury and, equally importantly, excluding injury by clinical examination is unreliable. The threshold for investigating blunt abdominal trauma should, therefore, be low.[3,4] This applies particularly in patients who have been sedated, and those with a decreased level of consciousness, whether due to concomitant head injury or intoxication.[1,5,6,7] Confirmation of the presence or absence of blunt abdominal injury, therefore, relies largely on the use of diagnostic adjuncts.[8]

The success of non-operative treatment of solid organ injury, first pioneered by paediatric surgeons,[9] together with more accurate imaging and minimally invasive techniques of haemorrhage control, led to a paradigm shift in the management of abdominal injury. Although exsanguinating haemorrhage and hollow viscus injury still require rapid and skilled surgery, non-operative management has become the standard of care for most other injuries, and been shown to be safe and effective.[10–12] This trend has been paralleled by a change in imaging algorithms, with greater emphasis on the detection of specific findings, rather than the mere detection of intraperitoneal fluid, which does not predict the need for intervention.[8,13] Non-operative management has, however, also created new controversies, such as in the exclusion of hollow viscus injuries. The selection of appropriate investigations is, therefore, more important than ever.

The principal, first-line investigations available are ultrasonography and CT. These tests are complementary rather than interchangeable, and their utility depends on the clinical context. Plain abdominal radiography has no role in the assessment of blunt abdominal trauma, as abdominal X-rays do not visualise abdominal viscera or demonstrate free fluid and, therefore, cannot provide direct evidence of organ injury or indirect evidence of haemorrhage. Abdominal X-rays may provide indirect evidence of hollow viscus injury by demonstrating a pneumoperitoneum, but lack sensitivity and specificity in this context. Chest and pelvic X-rays continue to have an important role as adjuncts to the primary survey of trauma patients and may suggest haemorrhage in adjacent cavities, but also cannot rule out intra-abdominal bleeding or visceral injury.[8]

Key point 4

- Confirmation of the presence or absence of blunt abdominal injury relies largely on the use of diagnostic adjuncts.

APPROACHES TO INVESTIGATION

Haemodynamically unstable patients

The primary aim in haemodynamically unstable blunt trauma patients is to arrest haemorrhage.[8] If the source of haemorrhage is intra-abdominal, this will usually require laparotomy and investigation, therefore, only serves to localise the site of haemorrhage to the abdomen.[7,8] In this context, the investigation of choice is a limited ultrasound examination,[8,13,14] which can be performed quickly, and without moving the patient from the resuscitation area.[8] The only finding which furthers the patient's management in this context is the presence or absence of free fluid, which in trauma is assumed to be blood or gastrointestinal content. If free fluid is demonstrated, the patient should usually proceed to immediate laparotomy (Fig. 1).[7,8,15,16]

FAST (focused abdominal sonography for trauma) is an abbreviated, protocolised ultrasonographic examination whose only objective is to

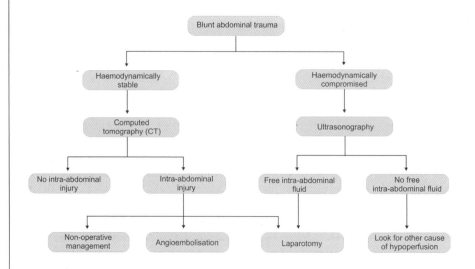

Fig. 1 Algorithm for the investigation and primary management of blunt abdominal trauma.

demonstrate intraperitoneal and pericardial fluid,[8] whereas a formal abdominal ultrasound, usually performed by a radiologist, also looks for signs of organ injury. Since the presence or absence of organ injury does not alter management in this setting, the temptation to perform lengthy examinations should be resisted. Several studies have shown FAST to be both sensitive and specific, particularly in haemodynamically-compromised patients,[17–20] although many early studies were marked by heterogeneity and, in particular, by the inclusion of both haemodynamically stable and unstable patients.

Key point 5

- In haemodynamically unstable patients, confirmation of intra-abdominal haemorrhage usually mandates laparotomy. A limited ultrasound examination, seeking free intra-abdominal fluid, which in the context trauma is assumed to be blood or gastro-intestinal content, is the investigation of choice in this setting.

Haemodynamically stable patients

The aims of investigation in haemodynamically stable patients differ. In contrast to patients with haemodynamic compromise, injuries require precise definition, as many will be amenable to non-operative management, and the decision to operate does not depend solely on the demonstration of a haemoperitoneum. This situation requires a test which is both sensitive and specific. FAST will miss injuries not associated with intra-abdominal fluid and, therefore, has no utility in haemodynamically stable patients, and even formal abdominal ultrasonography lacks the degree of sensitivity and specificity required in this context.[5,8,13] A recent review combining the results of eight major published series reported a sensitivity of 74% for organ injury.[8,13] The resulting consensus guideline concluded that ultrasound is not a satisfactory imaging modality for haemodynamically stable patients, because up to a quarter of hepatic and splenic injuries, most renal injuries, and virtually all pancreatic, mesenteric, bladder and gut injuries may be missed.[8,13] A separate meta-analysis reached similar conclusions,[21] and a Cochrane review analysing the use of ultrasound-based treatment algorithms, albeit also marred by heterogeneity, found no evidence in favour of ultrasonography in blunt trauma.[8,22]

The investigation of choice in haemodynamically stable patients is, therefore, CT (Fig. 1).[8,13,14] Its principal advantage is the ability to detect arterial contrast extravasation,[23] uncontained or as a pseudo-aneurysm, which predicts the need for surgery or angio-embolisation. Computed tomography also accurately evaluates the retroperitoneum, but is less sensitive for detecting hollow viscus injuries,[8,13] although detection rates are improving with increasing experience.[24] Computed tomography is also the modality of choice for diagnosing diaphragmatic injuries,[13] which may result in major morbidity and mortality if undetected, and may not present until many years after the event.[8]

Computed tomography, however, involves exposure to ionising radiation and intravenous contrast media. Furthermore, in most hospitals, CT requires movement of the patient away from the resuscitation area and is, therefore, not appropriate in haemodynamically compromised patients, although turnaround times are decreasing as a result of the trend towards locating scanners in or adjacent to emergency departments, and the proliferation of latest generation multi-detector helical scanners with faster image acquisition times.[8,25]

Key point 6

- Computed tomography is the investigation of choice in haemodynamically stable patients. Ultrasound lacks sensitivity and specificity in this setting.

Current controversies

The algorithm described above (Fig. 1) is widely practiced and accepted, but provoked fierce discussion when published recently as part of a review article in the *British Medical Journal*.[8] Several readers questioned the on-going use of ultrasound (formal or FAST) in the setting described, instead advocating the universal use of CT for all trauma patients, regardless of haemodynamic status. The superiority of CT is not in question, provided it can be performed safely and expeditiously, and faster scanners, ideally located close to or in resuscitation areas, have certainly contributed to an increasing proportion of patients undergoing CT rather than ultrasound examination. This development is entirely appropriate. The authors continue to believe strongly that there remains a small group of patients with profound and on-going haemodynamic compromise unresponsive to resuscitation, who (provided the source of the haemorrhage can be localised to the abdomen) belong in the operating room, and not the CT scanner. The decision as to whether a patient can safely be taken to the CT scanner, however, depends not only on the patient's condition, but also the time taken (transfer, acquisition, and review of images) to complete the scan. Achieving optimal timelines in this context requires a slick, experienced team familiar with working within the constrained environment of the scanner suite. Additional information, which CT will often provide, is useful, but surgeons providing trauma care must be prepared to proceed to laparotomy on the basis of an ultrasound, if operation is urgently required to control haemorrhage.

THE DIMINISHING ROLE OF DIAGNOSTIC PERITONEAL LAVAGE

Following its introduction in 1965, diagnostic peritoneal lavage rapidly became established as the standard of care, and remained so for several decades, until the advent of non-invasive imaging techniques. Diagnostic peritoneal lavage can be performed through an 'open' approach, similar to the Hassan technique for inserting a laparoscopic port, or using a percutaneous

Seldinger-type set. Once the catheter has been placed, any fluid present is aspirated. More than 10 ml of blood or the presence of gastrointestinal content is considered a frankly positive result and mandates laparotomy.[8] In the absence of these findings, a litre of warmed normal saline is infused into the peritoneal cavity, and then drained.[8] A sample of the effluent is submitted for laboratory examination.[8] The presence of > 100,000 red blood cells/mm^3 is regarded as indicative of a significant haemoperitoneum, whereas the presence of > 500 white cells/mm^3 or vegetable matter signifies a hollow viscus injury.[8] The presence of any of these parameters is regarded as an indication for laparotomy.[8]

A large, well-conducted, prospective study has shown diagnostic peritoneal lavage to be a highly accurate (sensitivity 95%, specificity 99%) test for intraperitoneal blood.[8,26] Diagnostic peritoneal lavage is also more sensitive than CT or ultrasound for the detection of hollow viscus injuries,[15] but does not exclude retroperitoneal injury.[8] Unlike ultrasound or CT, diagnostic peritoneal lavage is an invasive procedure and carries with it a small risk of visceral injury (0.6%).[26] Although, in principle, easy and quick to perform, this is not always the case, particularly in inexperienced hands, unco-operative or obese patients, and in those who have had previous abdominal surgery, and the need for microscopic analysis can delay further management.[8] The infusion of lavage fluid, which is never completely removed, may also interfere with the interpretation of subsequent imaging.[8]

Not all patients with a haemoperitoneum require laparotomy and by far the biggest drawback of diagnostic peritoneal lavage is a resulting high non-therapeutic laparotomy rate of up to 36%.[8,27] As a result, diagnostic peritoneal lavage is now much less commonly used in Europe and North America, where ultrasound has replaced it as the investigation of choice in haemodynamically unstable patients.[8,14,16,18] However, in resource-constrained environments, diagnostic peritoneal lavage is a useful technique for determining the presence of intraperitoneal blood, and it continues to have a role as a second-line investigation in the diagnosis of hollow viscus injuries.[8]

Key point 7

- As a primary investigation for blunt abdominal trauma in Western trauma centres, diagnostic peritoneal lavage is essentially obsolete.

FREE FLUID, BUT NO SOLID ORGAN INJURY, ON COMPUTED TOMOGRAPHY

Free intra-abdominal fluid without solid organ injury is a concern, particularly in neurologically compromised patients. In the majority, the fluid is blood, and of no further consequence; however, in around a quarter, the fluid is gastrointestinal content from an undetected hollow viscus injury.[29] A recent systematic review concluded that awake patients should be managed according to clinical examination findings, whereas neurologically compromised patients should undergo diagnostic peritoneal lavage to clarify the nature of the fluid.[8,29]

> **Key point 8**
>
> • The exclusion of hollow viscus injuries by imaging alone can be difficult.

PELVIC TRAUMA

The management of patients with pelvic fractures, particularly in the face of haemodynamic instability, remains contentious, and a detailed discussion is outwith the scope of this article. In broad terms, investigation should proceed along similar lines to other patients with major blunt abdominal trauma, albeit with attention to stabilisation of the pelvis.[8,30] Despite limitations, a recent systematic review[30] found in favour of FAST as the initial investigation of choice in haemodynamically compromised patients. Diagnostic peritoneal lavage in the presence of a pelvic fracture is associated with a high false-positive rate.[8] Haemodynamically stable patients with pelvic fractures should be evaluated by CT.[8,31]

WHAT IS THE NEGATIVE PREDICTIVE VALUE OF COMPUTED TOMOGRAPHY?

Patients without discernible injuries despite a significant mechanism are usually admitted to hospital for observation.[8] A systematic review has confirmed that a normal ultrasound scan does not exclude injury and should be followed by a period of observation, or further investigation.[7,13,21] In contrast, a large, prospective, multicentre study has shown that a normal abdominal CT scan has a high negative predictive value (99.63%), and concluded that admission for observation may not be necessary.[6] Such a strategy has obvious health economic appeal, but requires further study.[8]

STRATEGIES FOR MANAGEMENT

The complexity of abdominal injury management is the result of the almost infinite variety of possible injuries and combinations of injuries occurring in a diverse range of organ systems. Above all, treating such injuries requires sound decision-making. Although a detailed knowledge of the management of individual injuries is desirable, it is outwith the scope of this chapter, and less important than an appreciation of the different strategies for managing abdominal trauma. Such strategies form a spectrum, ranging from non-operative management, to minimally invasive techniques such as angio-embolisation, primary definitive surgery, and damage control surgery (Fig. 2).

NON-OPERATIVE MANAGEMENT OF SOLID ORGAN INJURY

The non-operative management of blunt splenic, hepatic and renal injury is well established. Criteria for attempting non-operative management include the absence of an associated injury necessitating laparotomy and haemodynamic stability. Approximately 60–80% of blunt splenic injuries[32] and 85–98% of hepatic injuries[33–35] can be managed non-operatively, with success

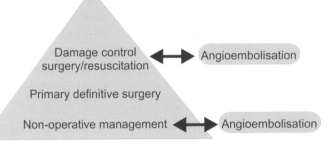

Fig. 2 Hierarchy of management strategies for management of blunt abdominal trauma.

rates approaching 95% (Fig. 3).[32] Non-operative management may be employed for all grades of splenic, hepatic and renal injury, but higher grades are associated with an increased failure rate and more complications.[32,36] The non-operative management of liver injuries is associated with higher morbidity than splenic injuries.[32] Delayed haemorrhage, hepatic abscess, biloma, and haemobilia are all recognised complications.[32]

Key point 9

- Many abdominal solid organ injuries can be managed non-operatively.

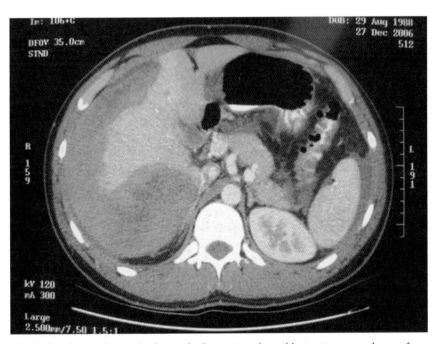

Fig. 3 Liver laceration and subcapsular/intraparenchymal haematoma, and some free fluid. Haemodynamically stable. Managed conservatively. Transfused 4 units of packed cells in total.

ANGIOGRAPHIC EMBOLISATION AS AN ADJUNCT TO NON-OPERATIVE MANAGEMENT

Angio-embolisation is increasingly used as an adjunct to the non-operative management of solid organ injury, particularly in haemodynamically stable patients with blunt splenic injuries,[37–40] hepatic injuries,[41] and renal injuries.[36,42,43] Although some authors have also advocated splenic angio-embolisation in transient responders to resuscitation,[44] such a strategy is risky and must be regarded with caution, as it probably only applies to a highly select subgroup of patients and, at present, few hospitals have the necessary resources for expeditious angiography and embolisation.[32] As a rule, haemodynamically unstable patients require laparotomy for arrest of haemorrhage, but the increasing trend towards interventional radiology operating theatres or operating angiography suites, which are fully equipped to provide both conventional surgical and minimally invasive approaches, will undoubtedly result in increased use of angio-embolisation for haemorrhage control.

Key point 10

• Angio-embolisation is a useful adjunct to non-operative management.

DAMAGE CONTROL RESUSCITATION AND DAMAGE CONTROL SURGERY

Damage control surgery is a strategy that sacrifices the completeness of the immediate repair in order to address the combined physiological impact of trauma and surgery.[45] It is arguably the most significant and far-reaching development in trauma management of the last three decades. The recognition that the restoration of physiology is paramount, and that lengthy operations exacerbate physiological derangement, led attempts to minimise operative time, in order to facilitate secondary resuscitation in the intensive care setting. This paradigm has since been developed further, largely as a result of experiences during the recent wars in South West Asia.[46] Increasing awareness of the need to manage the coagulopathy of trauma aggressively (haemostatic resuscitation) and integrating resuscitation and surgery has led to the introduction of the term 'damage control resuscitation', which emphasises the multimodal nature of this approach.[48] Damage control surgery forms part of this strategy, but must be used in the context of other interventions.

Surgical haemostasis should be viewed as an extension of managing the 'lethal triad' of acidosis, hypothermia, and coagulopathy. Severe haemorrhage precipitates an acute coagulopathy, probably through a hypoperfusion-mediated pathway, which is associated with significantly increased mortality.[48–51] Metabolic acidosis is the result of a switch to anaerobic metabolism and, therefore, lactate production due to hypoperfusion. Hypothermia is the consequence of both anaerobic metabolism, which limits endogenous heat production, and environmental exposure and administration of cold blood products and fluids.[52]

Key point 11

- Severe haemorrhage leads to coagulopathy, metabolic acidosis, and hypothermia (known as the 'lethal triad').

Obtaining control of haemorrhage is a crucial part of interrupting the ensuing vicious cycle but, in the presence of profound metabolic and haematological abnormalities, requires a different approach to other types of emergency surgery. Damage control surgery encompasses a range of techniques, such as abdominal packing, shunting of vascular injuries, and gastrointestinal resection without anastomosis, to stop bleeding, and limit contamination, in order to minimise the metabolic impact of treatment.

However, operative treatment must proceed in tandem with resuscitation, and the management of traumatic coagulopathy in particular is undergoing dramatic changes at the moment. Several recent retrospective studies have shown that the liberal use of fresh frozen plasma, irrespective of the results of clotting assays, is associated with improved survival,[53–55] and many authorities now recommend transfusion of packed cells, fresh frozen plasma, and even platelets, in equal proportions, in the most critically injured. Although promising, the evidence for such strategies is still weak and, therefore, remains controversial. Furthermore, obtaining supplies of valuable blood products, without prior laboratory evidence of coagulopathy remains a considerable practical challenge in UK practice.

Key point 12

- Damage control resuscitation is a multimodal strategy for the restoration of normal physiology, consisting of haemostatic resuscitation and rapid surgical haemostasis.

ANGIOGRAPHIC EMBOLISATION AS AN ADJUNCT TO DAMAGE CONTROL SURGERY

Several groups have also demonstrated the utility of angiographic embolisation as an adjunct to damage control surgery.[41,56–58] The management of patients with complex hepatic injuries in particular, which are often diagnosed intra-operatively in patients who required immediate laparotomy for profound haemodynamic compromise, may benefit from this strategy. Perihepatic packing is used to control parenchymal bleeding, followed by angiography and embolisation to obtain control of hepatic arterial injuries (Fig. 4). Again, this approach necessitates suitable and readily available angiography facilities, ideally in a combined operating/ interventional radiology theatre, which unfortunately remains aspirational in most UK hospitals.

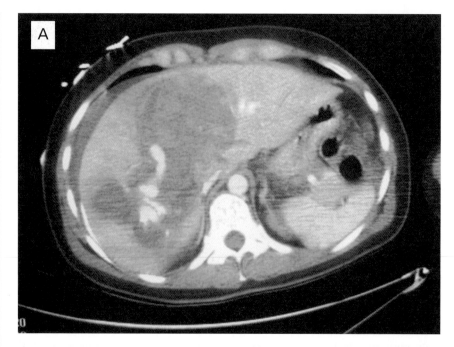

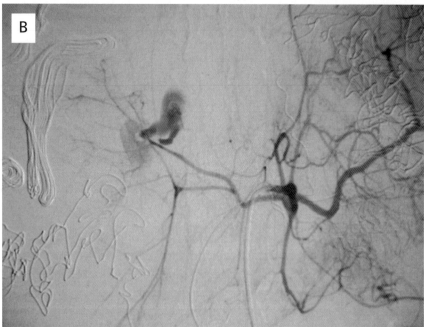

Fig. 4 (A) Intraparenchymal haematoma with active extravasation of contrast. Patient proceeded to laparotomy because of rapid deterioration in haemodynamic condition. Intra-operatively, a complex hepatic injury with central arterial haemorrhage was diagnosed and managed with perihepatic packing and temporary abdominal closure, followed by immediate transfer to the angiography suite for embolisation on completion of procedure. (B) Angiography confirmed bleeding from a branch of the hepatic artery, which was embolised. Note the abdominal packs around the liver. (C) Appearances following embolisation. The patient survived.

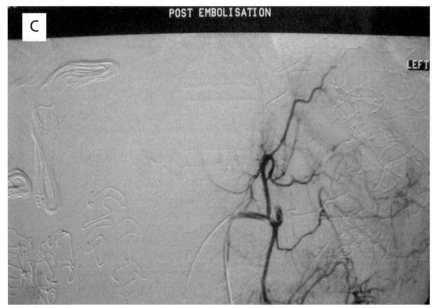

Fig. 4 C

PRIMARY DEFINITIVE SURGERY

Damage control surgery is resource intensive and associated with considerable potential morbidity; it must, therefore, be employed judiciously. Most abdominal injuries necessitating operative intervention can be managed with primary definitive surgery, and the damage control approach should be reserved for the most severely injured only.

Key point 13

- Primary definitive surgery is appropriate in the majority of patients requiring operative treatment.

CONCLUSIONS

Both the investigation and management of blunt abdominal trauma have undergone marked changes in recent years. CT is the investigation of choice, but ultrasound remains a useful tool for the diagnosis of intra-abdominal haemorrhage in the critically unstable patient. Diagnostic peritoneal lavage has become virtually obsolete.

Non-operative management of solid organ injury has become the standard of care in haemodynamically stable patients in whom hollow viscus injury can be excluded with reasonable confidence. Interventional radiology is likely to play an ever increasing role, and the distinction between resuscitation room, operating theatre, CT scanner, and angiography suite will become increasingly blurred in the future. Similarly, as an increasing proportion of patients are managed without surgery, treatment will be provided by intensivists and radiologists, and the surgeon's role will change to co-ordination of management. Despite these developments, a small number of patients with catastrophic intra-abdominal injuries will continue to require immediate and skilled surgical intervention combined with expert resuscitation. Such injuries require a different approach to other types of emergency surgery, and should ideally be managed by surgeons and anaesthetists with an interest and experience in this area.

Key points for clinical practice

- Blunt intra-abdominal injury results from direct compression or deceleration.

- Extra-abdominal injury is important in identifying the risk of abdominal injury.

- Diagnosing and excluding intra-abdominal injury by clinical examination is unreliable, particularly in patients with a decreased level of consciousness.

- Confirmation of the presence or absence of blunt abdominal injury relies largely on the use of diagnostic adjuncts.

- In haemodynamically unstable patients, confirmation of intra-abdominal haemorrhage usually mandates laparotomy. A limited ultrasound examination, seeking free intra-abdominal fluid, which in the context trauma is assumed to be blood or gastro-intestinal content, is the investigation of choice in this setting.

- Computed tomography is the investigation of choice in haemodynamically stable patients. Ultrasound lacks sensitivity and specificity in this setting.

- As a primary investigation for blunt abdominal trauma in Western trauma centres, diagnostic peritoneal lavage is essentially obsolete.

- The exclusion of hollow viscus injuries by imaging alone can be difficult.

- Many abdominal solid organ injuries can be managed non-operatively.

- Angio-embolisation is a useful adjunct to non-operative management.

- Severe haemorrhage leads to coagulopathy, metabolic acidosis, and hypothermia (known as the 'lethal triad').

- Damage control resuscitation is a multimodal strategy for the restoration of normal physiology, consisting of haemostatic resuscitation and rapid surgical haemostasis.

- Primary definitive surgery is appropriate in the majority of patients requiring operative treatment.

References

1. National Confidential Enquiry into Perioperative Deaths. *Trauma: Who Cares?* London: NCEPOD, 2007.
2. Gilroy D. Deaths from blunt trauma, after arrival at hospital: plus ça change, plus c'est la même chose. *Injury* 2005; **36**: 47–50.
3. Hoff WS, Holevar M, Nagy KK *et al.*; Eastern Association for the Surgery of Trauma. Practice management guidelines for the evaluation of blunt abdominal trauma: the EAST practice management guidelines work group. *J Trauma* 2002; **53**: 602–615.
4. Salim A, Sangthong B, Martin M, Brown C, Plurad D, Demetriades D. Whole body imaging in blunt multisystem trauma patients without obvious signs of injury. *Arch Surg* 2006; **141**: 468–475.
5. Myers J. Focused assessment with sonography for trauma (FAST): the truth about ultrasound in blunt trauma. *J Trauma* 2007; **62**: S28.
6. Livingston DH, Lavery RF, Passannante MR *et al.* Admission or observation is not necessary after a negative abdominal computed tomographic scan in patients with suspected blunt abdominal trauma: results of a prospective, multi-institutional trial. *J Trauma* 1998; **44**: 273–280.
7. Isenhour JL, Marx J. Advances in abdominal trauma. *Emerg Med Clin North Am* 2007; **25**: 713–733.
8. Jansen JO, Yule SR, Loudon MA. Investigation of blunt abdominal trauma. *BMJ* 2008; **336**; 938–942.
9. Upadhyaya P, Simpson JS. Splenic trauma in children. *Surg Gynaecol Obstet* 1968; **126**: 781–790.
10. Velmahos GC, Toutouzas KG, Radin R, Chan L, Demetriades D. Nonoperative management of blunt injury to solid abdominal organs: a prospective study. *Arch Surg* 2003; **138**: 844–851.
11. Haan JM, Bocchicchio GV, Kramer N, Scalea TM. Nonoperative management of blunt splenic injury: a 5-year experience. *J Trauma* 2005; **58**: 492–498.
12. Stein DM, Scalea TM. Nonoperative management of spleen and liver injuries. *J Intensive Care Med* 2006; **21**: 296–304.
13. Shuman WP, Holtzman SR, Bree RL *et al.* American College of Radiology Appropriateness Criteria. Blunt Abdominal Trauma. 2005 <http://www.acr.org/SecondaryMainMenuCategories/quality_safety/app_criteria/pdf/ExpertPanelonGastrointestinalImaging.aspx> [Accessed 20 November 2007].
14. The Royal College of Radiologists. Making the best use of clinical radiology services: referral guidelines. London: The Royal College of Radiologists, 2007.
15. Hoff WS, Holevar M, Nagy KK *et al.*; Eastern Association for the Surgery of Trauma. Practice management guidelines for the evaluation of blunt abdominal trauma: the EAST practice management guidelines work group. *J Trauma* 2002; **53**: 602–615.
16. Scalea T, Rodriguez A, Chiu W *et al.* Focused assessment with sonography for trauma (FAST): results from an International Consensus Conference. *J Trauma* 1999; **46**: 466–472.
17. Healey M, Simons RK, Winchell RJ *et al.* A prospective evaluation of abdominal ultrasound in trauma: is it useful? *J Trauma* 1996; **40**: 875–885.
18. Boulanger BR, McLellan BA, Brenneman FD *et al.* Emergent abdominal sonography as a screening test in a new diagnostic algorithm for blunt trauma. *J Trauma* 1996; **40**: 867–874.
19. Rozycki GS, Ochsner MG, Jaffin JH, Champion HR. Prospective evaluation of surgeons' use of ultrasound in the evaluation of trauma patients. *J Trauma* 1993; **34**: 516–527.
20. Rozycki GS, Ballard RB, Feliciano DV, Schmidt JA, Pennington SD. Surgeon-performed ultrasound for the assessment of truncal injuries: lessons learned from 1540 patients. *Ann Surg* 1998; **228**: 557–567.
21. Stengel D, Bauwens K, Sehouli J *et al.* Systematic review and meta-analysis of emergency ultrasonography for blunt abdominal trauma. *Br J Surg* 2001; **88**: 901–912.
22. Stengel D, Bauwens K, Sehouli J *et al.* Emergency-ultrasound-based algorithms for diagnosing blunt abdominal trauma. *Cochrane Database Syst Rev* 2005; (2): CD004446.
23. Yao DC, Jeffrey RB, Mirvis SE *et al.* Using contrast-enhanced helical CT to visualize arterial extravasation after blunt abdominal trauma: incidence and organ distribution. *AJR Am J Roentgenol* 2002; **178**: 17–20.

24. Brody JM, Leighton DB, Murphy BL *et al*. CT of blunt trauma bowel and mesenteric injury: typical findings and pitfalls in diagnosis. *Radiographics* 2000; **20**: 1525–1536.

25. Shanmuganathan K. Multi-detector row CT imaging of blunt abdominal trauma. *Semin Ultrasound CT MR* 2004; **25**: 180–124.

26. Nagy KK, Roberts RR, Joseph KT *et al*. Experience with over 2500 diagnostic peritoneal lavages. *Injury* 2000; **31**: 479–482.

27. Bain IM, Kirby RM, Tiwari P *et al*. Survey of abdominal ultrasound and diagnostic peritoneal lavage for suspected intra-abdominal injury following blunt trauma. *Injury* 1998; **29**: 65–71.

28. Boulanger BR, Kearney PA, Brenneman FD, Tsuei B, Ochoa J. Utilization of FAST (focused assessment with sonography for trauma) in 1999: results of a Survey of North American Trauma Centers. *Am Surg* 2000; **65**: 1049–1055.

29. Rodriguez C, Barone JE, Wilbanks TO, Rha CK, Miller K. Isolated free fluid on computed tomographic scan in blunt abdominal trauma: a systematic review of incidence and management. *J Trauma* 2002; **53**: 79–85.

30. Heetveld MJ, Harris I, Schlaphoff G, Sugrue M. Guidelines for the management of haemodynamically unstable pelvic fracture patients. *Aust NZ J Surg* 2004; **74**: 520–529.

31. Heetveld MJ, Harris I, Schlaphoff G, Balogh Z, D'Amours SK, Sugrue M. Hemodynamically unstable pelvic fractures: recent care and new guidelines. *World J Surg* 2004; **28**: 904–909.

32. Schroeppel TJ, Croce MA. Diagnosis and management of blunt abdominal solid organ injury. *Curr Opin Crit Care* 2007; **13**: 399–404.

33. Velmahos GC, Toutouzas K, Radin R *et al*. High success with nonoperative management of blunt hepatic trauma: the liver is a sturdy organ. *Arch Surg* 2003; **138**: 475–481.

34. Croce MA, Fabian TC, Menke PG *et al*. Nonoperative management of blunt hepatic trauma is the treatment of choice for hemodynamically stable patients results of a prospective trial. *Ann Surg* 1995; **221**: 744–755.

35. Malhotra AK, Fabian TC, Croce MA *et al*. Blunt hepatic injury: a paradigm shift from operative to nonoperative management in the 1990s. *Ann Surg* 2000; **231**: 804–813.

36. Santucci RA, Wessels H, Bartsch G *et al*. Evaluation and management of renal injuries: consensus statement of the renal trauma subcommittee. *Br J Urol* 2004; **93**: 937–954.

37. Haan JM, Bochicchio GV, Jurkovich GJ. Non-operative management of blunt splenic injury: a 5-year experience. *J Trauma* 2005; **58**: 492–498.

38. Bee TK, Croce MA, Miller PR, Pritchard FE, Davis KA, Fabian TC. Failures of splenic nonoperative management: is the glass half empty or half full? *J Trauma* 2001; **50**: 230–236.

39. Davis KA, Fabian TC, Croce MA *et al*. Improved success in nonoperative management of blunt splenic injuries: embolization of splenic artery pseudoaneurysms. *J Trauma* 1998; **44**: 1008–1015.

40. Wei B, Hemmila MR, Arbabi S, Taheri PA, Wahl WL. Angioembolization reduces operative intervention for blunt splenic injury. *J Trauma* 2008; **64**: 1472–1477.

41. Gaarder C, Naess PA, Eken T *et al*. Liver injuries – improved results with a formal protocol including angiography. *Injury* 2007; **38**: 1075–1083.

42. Hagiwara A, Sakaki S, Goto H *et al*. The role of interventional radiology in the management of blunt renal injury: a practical protocol. *J Trauma* 2001; **51**: 526–531.

43. Sofocleous CT, Hinrichs C, Hubbi B *et al*. Angiographic findings and embolotherapy in renal arterial trauma. *Cardiovasc Intervent Radiol* 2005; **28**: 39–47.

44. Hagiwara A, Murata A, Matsuda T, Matsuda H, Shimazaki S. The usefulness of transcatheter arterial embolization for patients with blunt polytrauma showing transient response to fluid resuscitation. *J Trauma* 2004; **57**: 271–277.

45. Loveland JA, Boffard KD. Damage control in the abdomen and beyond. *Br J Surg* 2004; **91**: 1095–1101.

46. Holcomb JB, Jenkins D, Rhee P *et al*. Damage control resuscitation: directly addressing the early coagulopathy of trauma. *J Trauma* 2007; **62**: 307–310.

47. Hodgetts TJ, Mahoney PF, Kirkman E. Damage control resuscitation. *J R Army Med Corps* 2007; **153**: 299–300.

48. Brohi K, Cohen MJ, Ganter MT *et al*. Acute coagulopathy of trauma: hypoperfusion induces systemic anticoagulation and hyperfibrinolysis. *J Trauma* 2008; **64**: 1211–1217.

49. Brohi K, Singh J, Heron M, Coats T. Acute traumatic coagulopathy. *J Trauma* 2003; **54**: 1127–1130.
50. MacLeod JB, Lynn M, McKenney MG *et al.* Early coagulopathy predicts mortality in trauma. *J Trauma* 2003; **55**: 39–44.
51. Wang HE, Callaway CW, Peitzman AB, Tisherman SA. Admission hypothermia and outcome after major trauma. *Crit Care Med* 2005; **33**: 1296–1301.
52. Schreiber MA. Coagulopathy in the trauma patient. *Curr Opin Crit Care* 2005; **11**: 590–597.
53. Gunter OL, Au BK, Isbell JM, Mowery NT, Young PP, Cotton BA. Optimizing outcomes in damage control resuscitation: identifying blood product ratios associated with improved survival. *J Trauma* 2008; **65**: 527–534.
54. Cotton BA, Gunter OL, Isbell J *et al.* Damage control haematology: the impact of a trauma exsanguination protocol on survival and blood product utilization. *J Trauma* 2008; **64**: 1177–1183.
55. Duchesne JC, Hunt JP, Wahl G *et al.* Review of current blood transfusions strategies in a mature level I trauma center: were we wrong for the last 60 years? *J Trauma* 2008; **65**: 272–278.
56. Johnson J, Gracias VH, Gupta R *et al.* Hepatic angiography in patients undergoing damage control laparotomy. *J Trauma* 2002; **52**: 1102–1106.
57. Asensio JA, Demetriades D, Chahwan S *et al.* Approach to the management of complex hepatic injuries. *J Trauma* 2000; **48**: 66–69.
58. Asensio JA, Roldan G, Petrone P *et al.* Operative management and outcomes in 103 AAST-OIS grades IV and V complex hepatic injuries: trauma surgeons still need to operate, but angioembolization helps. *J Trauma* 2003; **54**: 647–654.

Peter McCulloch

9

Minimally invasive gastrectomy and oesophagectomy

Minimally invasive surgery has developed in a somewhat unpredictable fashion over the last 10 years which has clearly illustrated the problems of developing evidence for new surgical techniques. Some techniques, like splenectomy, have become routine, whilst the barriers to developing randomised trials for surgical operations have frustrated the development of evidence and produced a confusing morass of uncontrolled studies with disparate and poorly defined outcomes both for good and ill. Minimally invasive gastrectomy and oesophagectomy for cancer are both now increasing in popularity, but neither has become widely accepted, as yet, in the West, and the evidence of benefit for either must still be regarded as inconclusive. The development of the two operations has been quite different technically and geographically, for reasons related to the nature of the patient populations. The argument that minimal trauma to the well-innervated body wall must be a good thing is so persuasive that efforts to demonstrate clinical benefit will no doubt continue. Whether these can be reconciled with demands for tight regulation of new procedures to ensure patient safety, or with the need to produce convincing scientific evidence, remains to be seen.

GASTRECTOMY

HISTORY

The history of laparoscopic gastrectomy is fairly short, and much more straightforward than that of oesophagectomy. The first published report of a laparoscopic distal gastrectomy, by Peter Goh and colleagues, appeared in 1992,[1] and the first gastrectomies for cancer were reported in 1995.[2,3] The first

Peter McCulloch MBChB MA MD FRCS(Ed) FRCS(Glas)
Clinical Reader in Surgery, Nuffield Department of Surgery, University of Oxford, John Radcliffe Hospital, Headley Way, Headington, Oxford OX3 9DU, UK. E-mail: peter.mcculloch@nds.ox.ac.uk

completely laparoscopic total gastrectomy and the first reports incorporating extended (D2) radical lymphadenectomy were in 1999.[4,5]

DEVELOPMENT

A systematic review conducted in 2006 found reports relating to over 2500 cases world-wide, excluding case reports and reports of less than six cases.[6] A recent update I conducted recorded reports of over 3000 further cases. There is a very striking Eastern predominance in the literature, illustrated by two recent multicentre studies from Japan and Korea, each documenting more than 1200 cases.[7,8] Western reports, by contrast, have been much smaller in numbers and generally less adventurous technically. The accelerating trend towards minimally invasive surgery can be partly attributed to technical improvements which have reduced some of the difficulties associated with the minimally invasive approach. The key development was the invention of the harmonic scalpel and similar microwave energy devices for haemostatically secure dissection, but major advances in stapler technology and improved optics have also been important.

The different patterns of development in East and West are interesting. Minimally invasive surgery has become widely practiced in Japan and Korea in particular, but tends still to be restricted to cases of early cancer. D2 lymph node dissection has been reported from numerous centres in these countries in the last 5 years, and is clearly feasible and safe in these settings. Several centres are engaged in studies to evaluate the use of sentinel node biopsy with minimally invasive surgery, and there have been reports of technical advances such as proximal gastrectomy with Merendino interposition, vagus and pylorus sparing gastrectomy and the use of a semi-flexible endoscope. However, total gastrectomy remains a relative rarity, and the majority of surgeons still favour a hand-assisted Billroth I anastomosis performed through a small mid-line incision. The high frequency of early diagnosis of disease in these countries and the very low mortality of open D2 surgery have probably influenced the restriction of minimally invasive surgery to early cancer, whilst the comfort of most surgeons with D2 dissection from early in their training, and the striking lack of intra-abdominal fat in Eastern patients may have encouraged the adoption of D2 minimally invasive surgery and of sentinel node biopsy. The use of the mini-laparotomy reflects the anatomical differences between East and West: the anteroposterior depth of the abdominal cavity is strikingly less in the average East Asian patient than in Western Europeans, and the stomach is a longer narrower organ, making Billroth I anastomosis through a small incision without tension feasible in most cases of distal cancer.

In the West, the challenges are different: the *Helicobacter pylori* epidemic and its' accidental eradication[9] have resulted in declining numbers of distal cancers in an ever-older cohort of patients. With less opportunities to progress along their learning curve, Western surgeons have been less adventurous than those in the East, with few series of D2 dissection or total gastrectomy. At the same time, they have explored the use of minimally invasive gastrectomy in the frail and elderly where no potentially curative alternative exists.[10] This has highlighted another major inhibitory factor for the development of minimally invasive gastrectomy in the West, namely strong ethical and regulatory concerns in some countries, which make surgeons very cautious about performing unconventional procedures which carry any risk of mortality, even if no viable alternative treatment exists.

> ## Key points 1
>
> - Differences in the speed and direction of development of minimally invasive gastrectomy in East and West reflect the anatomical differences in the patient population and the much greater detection frequency of early cancer in the East.

TECHNIQUE

The basics of minimally invasive gastrectomy technique are now well established and relatively invariant. Between 3 and 5 ports are used in the upper half of the abdomen, with the liver retracted by a Nathanson or fan retractor (or remarkably, in Japan, by transfixion and retraction with a single large suture through the abdominal wall!). Most surgeons, even in Japan, do not attempt the traditional D2 dissection of the omentum and anterior leaf of the mesocolon *en bloc*, since it is much quicker to divide the gastrocolic omentum or separate it from the colon. The first major vessels ligated are the right gastro-epiploics on the antero-inferior surface of the pancreas, and the duodenum is stapled across either at this point or after opening the lesser omentum and dividing the right gastric vessels. After identifying and dividing the left gastro-epiploic vessels, the D2 nodal dissection is performed along the hepatic and splenic arteries before isolating and dividing the left gastric vein and artery individually. Most surgeons clip the large named vessels, and some also suture the left gastric artery. Dissection of the lesser curve and application of successive Endo-staplers completes the resection. Reconstruction differs in East and West as noted. Western surgeons normally use a fully laparoscopic approach to form a Billroth II anastomosis or a Roux-Y reconstruction.

The additional dissection for total gastrectomy is not problematic, but the oesophagojejunal anastomosis is, as shown by the numerous variants which have been proposed. The other common areas of subjective technical difficulty in minimally invasive gastrectomy are, in the order they are encountered, identification and clipping of the right gastro-epiploic vessels at their base, clearance of the duodenum for division, and identification of (and access to)

> ## Key point 2
>
> - The main areas of technical difficulty in minimally invasive gastrectomy using current techniques are: (i) the anastomosis for total gastrectomy; (ii) identification and division of the right gastro-epiploic vessels; and (iii) identification and division of the left gastric vessels.

the left gastric vessels. All of these can be very easy in a small, slim patient and very taxing in a large obese one. Flopping of the stomach and greater omentum into the field of view is sometimes very troublesome. Finally, where D2 dissection is carried out, entry into, and maintenance of, the correct retroperitoneal plane is important and difficult in the obese.

EVIDENCE BASE

Currently, minimally invasive gastrectomy is an excellent example of one of the most important unsolved problems for surgery: how to provide good quality valid evidence for new surgical procedures. The difficulties of performing randomised trials of surgical techniques have been analysed by many authors,[11,12] and some are significant and difficult to overcome. Unfortunately, surgeons have not proved terribly interested in developing 'next best' alternatives suited to the realities of technical development in their discipline. Alternatives such as the conversion of registries into prospective collaborative 'Phase IIS' studies have been proposed but have yet to be widely adopted. Instead, we have, in the case of minimally invasive gastrectomy, a profusion of case series reported in idiosyncratic and often incompatible ways, with the resultant huge difficulties in interpretation. Selection and publication biases are evident in the skewing of the literature towards excellent results. There have been some attempts to examine learning curves[13,14] and to provide meaningful non-randomised comparisons, and there have been at least three small randomised trials of distal gastrectomy.[15–17] Each of these has reported the results of a single surgeon, so their general applicability is doubtful. What the data reported show is that minimally invasive surgery is consistently associated with smaller operative blood loss, and faster return of gastrointestinal function than open resection in contemporary reports in similar settings; surprisingly, the evidence on hospital stay is inconsistent and unclear. Minimally invasive surgery generally appears very safe, although some smaller reports, presumably including the early learning curve, show alarming mortality and complication rates, with unusual types of complication not normally seen in open surgery. It is also notable that the anastomotic leak rate in the pooled data is unfeasibly low, given that there is no good reason to expect laparoscopic anastomoses to be more secure than open ones: this is almost certainly due to selection and reporting bias. Whether minimally invasive surgery is as satisfactory a cancer operation as open surgery is not yet established. The pooled data from Western studies show a very unsatisfactory average yield of 10 nodes per operation, whilst Eastern studies showed 3 times that number[6] (*Note:* these figures were incorrectly transposed in the published version of the review). The evidence was not good enough for any sensible evaluation of the risk of involved resection margins, although in theory the loss of tactile sensation would increase this risk where the tumour cannot be clearly seen. My own judgement is that the Western figures reflect the limited experience in Western countries and the nature of the patients operated on, and that, as with open radical gastrectomy, Western surgeons will eventually be able to reproduce Eastern results with appropriate training and experience.

THE FUTURE

The challenges for the next few years are to develop and diffuse expertise so that the ability to perform D2 dissection and total gastrectomy by minimally invasive gastrectomy becomes less scattered, and to conduct valid studies to establish the real short- and long-term outcomes. The technical challenges involved in these procedures will hopefully engender innovations and developments to remove the frustrations they currently cause. There are now at least three reports of robotic gastrectomy using the Da Vinci machine,[18–20] and this may become of interest if further studies show any evidence of potential benefit. There has been strong advocacy of the argument that minimally invasive surgery cannot achieve its potential without an accelerated recovery programme,[21] and these claims need to be evaluated.

Key point 3

- The current evidence is mostly of poor scientific quality, and is not adequate to confirm unequivocally any outcome advantage of minimally invasive gastrectomy over open operation.

OESOPHAGECTOMY

HISTORY

The first report of a series of thoracoscopic mobilisations of the oesophagus was in 1993[22] and the first totally minimally invasive operation was reported in 1999 by Watson et al.[23] Dexter et al.[24] reported the first thoracoscopic radical node dissection in the chest in 1996.

DEVELOPMENT

Since these pioneering studies, the popularity of the minimally invasive oesophagectomy technique has grown rather less rapidly than that of gastrectomy: in 2006 there were about 1400 reported cases contained in case series world-wide,[6] and an update to 2008 reveals about an additional 600 (although multiple update reports from some centres make assessment of numbers difficult). Compared to gastrectomy, the striking differences for minimally invasive oesophagectomy are: (i) the plethora of competing approaches and techniques; (ii) the Western dominance of the literature; and (iii) the continuing uncertainty over the safety of the technique.

Key points 4

- Minimally invasive oesophagectomy has been performed considerably less often than minimally invasive gastrectomy suggesting that the procedure may be more technically challenging.

Unlike gastrectomy, oesophagectomy necessarily invades both the chest and abdomen, and the possibilities for combining open and endoscopic approaches are, therefore, multiplied – and just about all of them have been tried. The most popular options appear to be laparoscopic gastric mobilisation with right thoracotomy, laparoscopic gastric mobilisation with transhiatal dissection of the mediastinum and cervical anastomosis, and combined thoracoscopic and laparoscopic dissection with the anastomosis either in the neck or chest. An additional complication has been the use of the prone position for thoracoscopic dissection, which appears, in some hands, to allow more rapid dissection and excellent short-term results.[25] As with gastrectomy, there are isolated reports of the use of robotic surgery.[26]

Key points 5

- There are multiple reported technical approaches for oesophagectomy, with no good comparative data or clear consensus on their relative merits.

There have been no randomised trials of minimally invasive oesophagectomy to date; although some comparisons against open surgery have been attempted, most of these have been too flawed in design to allow any clear evaluation of potential benefits of the technique. The literature has been dominated by the work of Jim Luketich and his team in Pittsburgh, whose series of (now) over 500 procedures is by far the largest in the world.[27] Their results are undoubtedly impressive, but their patients are clearly different from the average profile of oesophagectomy patients, and long-term outcomes are less clear than the short-term morbidity and mortality. Luketich's technique has developed over time, and currently consists of a laparoscopic gastric mobilisation followed by thoracoscopic mobilisation of the oesophagus through the right chest with the patient in the left lateral position, and an intrathoracic anastomosis. Luketich et al.[28] reported a mean hospital stay of 7 days, and a 1.4% mortality. The systematic review, on the other hand, showed an average mortality of 2.3%, and a hospital stay of over 11 days, not impressively different from that for open operation.[6] Operating times were usually over 5 h, and leak rates and conversion rates averaged around 8% and 5%, respectively. As with gastrectomy, the poor quality of the evidence makes interpretation very difficult, and the influence of publication and selection biases seems likely to be large. The disappointing figures over hospital stay suggest that the debilitating effects of large wounds may have been less important and those of mediastinal dissection more important than had previously been assumed. Currently, hopes of establishing convincing benefit over open surgery are focused on the recovery period after hospital discharge. The long-lasting impact of open oesophagectomy on function and symptoms has been extensively documented,[29] and there are early reports which give rise to hope that minimally invasive oesophagectomy may greatly reduce the time taken for patients to return to their pre-operative quality of life (unpublished data presented by Wajeed, Berrisford, Blazeby et al., AUGIS 2007).

Key points 6

- There is early evidence of a possible benefit in post-discharge quality of life after minimally invasive oesophagectomy: however, the current evidence is mostly of poor scientific quality, and is not adequate to confirm any outcome advantage of minimally invasive oesophagectomy over open operation.

Unlike gastrectomy, however, there are persistent reports of serious mortality and morbidity in minimally invasive oesophagectomy,[29,30] which have caused sufficient concerns to stop some programmes. The complications which have caused particular concern are unexplained respiratory failure with an ARDS picture in fit patients whose operation had apparently gone well, necrosis of the gastric tube and damage to the airway. All of these problems are highly lethal, and most unusual in open surgery. Whether they principally reflect inexperience or are more related to technical or physiological differences between the open and minimally invasive operations is currently impossible to say, although it is clear that the very experienced Pittsburgh unit has found ways of avoiding them.

Key points 7

- Anecdotal evidence of specific serious complications after minimally invasive oesophagectomy unusual in open oesophagectomy, such as tracheal damage or gastric tube necrosis, has caused concerns.

TECHNIQUE

Technically, the laparoscopic mobilisation of the stomach is very similar to a gastrectomy except that the right gastro-epiploic vessels are preserved with great care. The thoracoscopic approach with the patient in the left lateral position gives a view similar to that at Ivor Lewis oesophagectomy, but dissection of the mediastinum is made more difficult by lack of tactile sensation, particularly with reference to identifying and avoiding the airway. To assist with access to the lower pleura, various techniques have been devised to pull down the dome of the diaphragm. After this, the pleura is divided in the conventional manner, beginning with the inferior pulmonary ligament, and dividing the azygos vein early with a vascular stapler. Whilst it is technically feasible to perform a classical *en bloc* lower mediastinal clearance from the aortic adventitia forward, ligating the thoracic duct low in the chest and taking the subcarinal nodes, most surgeons do not. If the anastomosis is destined for the neck, freeing of the tissue at the apex of the chest cavity to allow the specimen to come up easily is important. Stapled anastomoses in the chest are done with a circular stapler introduced by enlarging one of the ports to a mini-thoracotomy. The head of the stapler may be introduced via this or per-orally. The prone position requires a considerable mental re-adjustment for surgeons used to the lateral view: one famous surgeon confesses he always writes on the theatre white board the acronym AC/DC (for 'aorta cranial – don't cut!). The advantage is that the lung falls away naturally allowing dissection without retraction, and sometimes allegedly without single-lung ventilation. Proponents claim it is quicker than conventional dissection, but the obvious concern is that, if serious bleeding was to occur, changing the position to allow emergency thoracotomy would be very difficult in the time available.

EVIDENCE BASE

The realities of specialist practice in the West mean that most upper gastrointestinal cancer surgeons now spend most of their time dealing with cancers of the lower oesophagus and O/G junction. These are challenging technically by any minimally invasive route, but reports to an independent confidential registry (MIMOCS, see <http://demo.e-dendrite.com/csp/migocs/frontpages/migocs.csp>) show that more surgeons are beginning to evaluate the minimally invasive approach. The lack of convincing evidence of benefit to date can justifiably be attributed to the early state of the learning curve for most units; as for gastrectomy, the surgical community needs to address the serious failings in its approach to evaluation and develop a more scientific approach to producing valid evidence of benefit. The operation remains a major undertaking whether open or not, and fear of criticism and possible sanction from governance authorities in the case of adverse outcomes has slowed development – whether for good or ill being a matter for speculation and debate. An agreed framework for producing meaningful evidence short of a randomised trial would be tremendously useful, particularly if regulatory authorities endorsed it and demanded that surgeons contribute to it until a better evaluation of the merits of the technique has been completed. In the meantime, the problem of how to ensure patient safety without inhibiting progress remains unresolved.

Key point 8

- Development towards a randomised trial would be facilitated by an intermediate stage of co-operative prospective data registration, to build consensus, define learning curves and allow power calculation estimates.

Key points for clinical practice

- Differences in the speed and direction of development of minimally invasive gastrectomy in East and West reflect the anatomical differences in the patient population and the much greater detection frequency of early cancer in the East.

Key points for clinical practice (continued)

- The main areas of technical difficulty in minimally invasive gastrectomy using current techniques are: (i) the anastomosis for total gastrectomy; (ii) identification and division of the right gastroepiploic vessels; and (iii) identification and division of the left gastric vessels.

- The current evidence is mostly of poor scientific quality, and is not adequate to confirm unequivocally any outcome advantage of minimally invasive gastrectomy over open operation.

- Minimally invasive oesophagectomy has been performed considerably less often than minimally invasive gastrectomy suggesting that the procedure may be more technically challenging.

- There are multiple reported technical approaches for oesophagectomy, with no good comparative data or clear consensus on their relative merits.

- There is early evidence of a possible benefit in post-discharge quality of life after minimally invasive oesophagectomy: however, the current evidence is mostly of poor scientific quality, and is not adequate to confirm any outcome advantage of minimally invasive oesophagectomy over open operation.

- Anecdotal evidence of specific serious complications after minimally invasive oesophagectomy unusual in open oesophagectomy, such as tracheal damage or gastric tube necrosis, has caused concerns.

- Development towards a randomised trial would be facilitated by an intermediate stage of co-operative prospective data registration, to build consensus, define learning curves and allow power calculation estmates.

References

1. Goh P, Tekant Y, Kum CK, Isaac J, Shang NS. Totally intra-abdominal laparoscopic Billroth II gastrectomy. *Surg Endosc* 1992; **6**: 160.
2. Watson DI, Devitt PG, Game PA. Laparoscopic Billroth II gastrectomy for early gastric cancer. *Br J Surg* 1995; **82**: 661–662.
3. Nagai Y, Tanimura H, Takifuji K, Kashiwagi H, Yamoto H, Nakatani Y. Laparoscope-assisted Billroth I gastrectomy. *Surg Laparosc Endosc* 1995; **5**: 281–287.
4. Uyama I, Sugioka A, Fujita J, Komori Y, Matsui H, Hasumi A. Laparoscopic total gastrectomy with distal pancreatosplenectomy and D2 lymphadenectomy for advanced gastric cancer. *Gastric Cancer* 1999; **2**: 230–234.
5. Azagra JS, Goergen M, De Simone P, Ibanez-Aguirre J. Minimally invasive surgery for gastric cancer. *Surg Endosc* 1999; **13**: 351–357.
6. Gemmill EH, McCulloch P. Systematic review of minimally invasive surgery for gastro-oesophageal cancer. *Br J Surg* 2007; **94**: 1461–1467.
7. Kurokawa Y, Katai H, Fukuda H, Sasako M; Gastric Cancer Surgical Study Group of the Japan Clinical Oncology Group. Phase II study of laparoscopy-assisted distal gastrectomy with nodal dissection for clinical stage I gastric cancer: Japan Clinical Oncology Group Study JCOG0703. *Jpn J Clin Oncol* 2008; **38**: 501–503.

8. Kim MC, Kim W, Kim HH *et al.*; Korean Laparoscopic Gastrointestinal Surgery Study (KLASS) Group. Risk factors associated with complication following laparoscopy-assisted gastrectomy for gastric cancer: a large-scale Korean multicenter study. *Ann Surg Oncol* 2008; **15**: 2692–2700.

9. Sipponen P. *Helicobacter pylori* gastritis – epidemiology. *J Gastroenterol* 1997; **32**: 273–277.

10. Singh KK, Rohatgi A, Rybinkina I, McCulloch P, Mudan S. Laparoscopic gastrectomy for gastric cancer: early experience among the elderly. *Surg Endosc* 2008; **22**: 1002–1007.

11. van der Linden W. On the generalization of surgical trial results. *Acta Chir Scand* 1980; **146**: 229–234.

12. McCulloch P, Taylor I, Sasako M, Lovett B, Griffin D. Randomised trials in surgery: problems and possible solutions. *BMJ* 2002; **324**: 1448–1451.

13. Kunisaki C, Makino H, Yamamoto N *et al.* Learning curve for laparoscopy-assisted distal gastrectomy with regional lymph node dissection for early gastric cancer. *Surg Laparosc Endosc Percutan Tech* 2008; **18**: 236–241.

14. Kim MC, Jung GJ, Kim HH. Learning curve of laparoscopy-assisted distal gastrectomy with systemic lymphadenectomy for early gastric cancer. *World J Gastroenterol* 2005; **11**: 7508–7511.

15. Huscher CG, Mingoli A, Sgarzini G *et al.* Laparoscopic versus open subtotal gastrectomy for distal gastric cancer: five-year results of a randomised prospective trial. *Ann Surg* 2005; **241**: 232–237.

16. Lee JH, San HS, Lee JH. A prospective randomized study comparing open vs laparoscopy-assisted distal gastrectomy in early gastric cancer. *Surg Endosc* 2005; **19**: 168–173.

17. Hayashi H, Ochiai T, Shimada H, Gunji Y. Prospective randomized study of open versus laparoscopy-assisted distal gastrectomy with extraperigastric lymph node dissection for early gastric cancer. *Surg Endosc* 2005; **19**: 1172–1176.

18. Anderson C, Ellenhorn J, Hellan M, Pigazzi A. Pilot series of robot-assisted laparoscopic subtotal gastrectomy with extended lymphadenectomy for gastric cancer. *Surg Endosc* 2007; **21**: 1662–1666.

19. Patriti A, Ceccarelli G, Bellochi R *et al.* Robot-assisted laparoscopic total and partial gastric resection with D2 lymph node dissection for adenocarcinoma. *Surg Endosc* 2008; **22**: 2753–2760.

20. Pugliese R, Maggioni D, Sansonna F *et al.* Outcomes and survival after laparoscopic gastrectomy for adenocarcinoma. Analysis on 65 patients operated on by conventional or robot-assisted minimal access procedures. *Eur J Surg Oncol* 2008 March 14 [Epub ahead of print].

21. Schulze S, Iversen MG, Bendixen A, Larsen TS, Kehlet H. Laparoscopic colonic surgery in Denmark 2004–2007. *Colorectal Dis* 2008; **10**: 869–870.

22. Gossot D, Fourquier P, Celerier M. Thoracoscopic esophagectomy: technique and initial results. *Ann Thorac Surg* 1993; **56**: 667–670.

23. Watson DI, Davies N, Jamieson GG. Totally endoscopic Ivor Lewis esophagectomy. *Surg Endosc* 1999; **13**: 293–297.

24. Dexter SP, Martin IG, McMahon MJ. Radical thoracoscopic esophagectomy for cancer. *Surg Endosc* 1996; **10**: 147–151.

25. Palanivelu C, Prakash A, Senthilkumar R *et al.* Minimally invasive esophagectomy: thoracoscopic mobilization of the esophagus and mediastinal lymphadenectomy in prone position–experience of 130 patients. *J Am Coll Surg* 2006; **203**: 7–16.

26. van Hillegersberg R, Boone J, Draaisma WA, Broeders IA, Giezeman MJ, Borel Rinkes IH. First experience with robot-assisted thoracoscopic esophagolymphadenectomy for esophageal cancer. *Surg Endosc* 2006; **20**: 1435–1439.

27. Nguyen NT, Gelfand D, Chang K *et al.* Laparoscopic esophagectomy. *Minerva Chir* 2005; **60**: 327–338.

28. Luketich JD, Alvelo-Rivera M, Buenaventura PO *et al.* Minimally invasive esophagectomy: outcomes in 222 patients. *Ann Surg* 2003; **238**: 486–494.

29. Conroy T, Marchal F, Blazeby JM. Quality of life in patients with oesophageal and gastric cancer: an overview. *Oncology* 2006; **70**: 391–402.

30. Atkins BZ, Fortes DL, Watkins KT. Analysis of respiratory complications after minimally invasive oesophagectomy: preliminary observation of persistent aspiration risk. *Dysphagia* 2007; **22**: 49–54.

James P. Byrne   David Mahon

10

Gastro-oesophageal reflux disease (GORD)

This chapter focuses on recent changes in our knowledge of reflux disease, epidemiology, current strategies for its management and emerging therapies being developed to manage this condition.

EPIDEMIOLOGY

Gastro-oesophageal reflux is a common foregut symptom, affecting up to half of the adult population, with the prevalence of oesophagitis possibly having doubled over a 10-year period.[1] A clear association between increasing body mass index and reflux disease has been described,[2] and it seems likely that this increase in prevalence of reflux disease is related to increasing levels of obesity.

Key point 1

• Reflux disease is increasing in prevalence, together with oesophageal adenocarcinoma and this may be mediated by increasing levels of obesity.

Increased frequency of transient lower oesophageal sphincter relaxation (TLESR) appears to be an important mechanism in the pathogenesis of gastro-oesophageal reflux disease and the mechanics of this have been elegantly described.[3] TLESRs have been found to be more common in obese subjects without symptoms of gastro-oesophageal reflux than controls[4] and this may explain how, if not why, reflux is more common in obese patients.

James Byrne BSc MBChB MD FRCS
Consultant General and Upper Gastrointestinal Surgeon, Southampton General Hospital, Tremona Road, Southampton SO16, UK. E-mail: james.byrne@suht.swest.nhs.uk

David Mahon MBChB MD FRCS(Gen)
Consultant Upper GI and Bariatric Surgeon, Musgrove Park NHS Trust, Taunton TA1 5DA, UK

It is now well-recognised that long-standing, severe, gastro-oesophageal reflux symptoms are strongly associated with development of oesophageal adenocarcinoma.[5] It is tempting, therefore, to speculate that the marked changes in incidence of oesophageal adenocarcinoma witnessed throughout the Western world over the last 30 years are, in part, a consequence of the well-documented increase in prevalence of obesity mediated by an increase in the incidence of chronic gastro-oesophageal reflux. It is not clear yet how the differing treatment strategies for managing reflux such as regular high-dose proton pump inhibitor, as-required intermittent proton pump inhibitor or anti-reflux surgery may modulate this risk of developing oesophageal adenocarcinoma.

DIAGNOSIS

Diagnosis of gastro-oesophageal reflux is often straightforward with typical symptoms of heartburn, regurgitation and dysphagia.

Reflux may also present with atypical symptoms such as non-cardiac chest pain or laryngopulmonary symptoms. Chronic cough and asthma are common in patients with reflux and patients may present without foregut symptoms to a wide variety of disciplines. Surgeons may be presented in clinic with patients in whom diagnosis and management decisions are particularly challenging. Patients may have been investigated by physicians with symptoms such as chest pain or shortness of breath that are attributed by them to a very large para-oesophageal hernia. Precise definition of the origin of upper gastrointestinal, cardiac and respiratory symptoms hernia is very important (but often difficult) in order that decisions regarding possible surgery are appropriately informed. Decisions in such complex patients are often best made following joint assessment with the relevant cardiologist or respiratory physician.

INVESTIGATION

Upper gastrointestinal endoscopy is mandatory in the pre-operative workup of patients prior to surgery. Pre-operative oesophageal manometry and 24-h pH study have been considered by many to be mandatory, although in the context of typical symptoms, response to proton pump inhibitor(PPI) therapy, and endoscopic findings confirming reflux-related oesophageal injury, many surgeons would not now consider pH monitoring to be essential. The Bravo™ wireless capsule system is a recent development that permits pH recording to be carried out without a wire connecting the pH probe to the recording device, and is generally much better tolerated by patients. The pH recording device is positioned in the lower oesophagus by means of a delivery device that is passed either orally or trans-nasally, and secured in position by a combination of suction and firing a locking pin which attaches the device to the mucosa. The device detaches itself after a period of time and passes thought the gut. As the device is generally very well-tolerated, patients are more likely to carry out their normal daily activities during the test, which may improve the accuracy of the investigation, and it is also possible to conduct studies over a period of 48–72 h.

Impedance monitoring has been in development for several years, and appears to have an important role in the management of patients with atypical symptoms together with those in whom symptoms are refractory to treatment with a proton pump inhibitor. It detects both liquid and gaseous episodes of reflux by measuring conductivity between electrodes placed at several levels throughout the oesophagus, and is generally combined with pH monitoring. Oesophageal impedance monitoring allows detection of the flow of liquids and gas up the oesophagus and permits discrimination between episodes of acid and non-acid reflux (*e.g.* bile reflux). It appears to be particularly useful in the investigation of patients with PPI-resistant reflux symptoms, chronic unexplained cough, and excessive belching, although its use is at present not wide-spread.[6] Prospective evaluation of 150 patients having anti-reflux surgery found intraluminal impedance pH monitoring to facilitate better patient selection for surgery than conventional pH monitoring alone.[7] In clinical practice, intraluminal impedance monitoring can be of great help in decision-making amongst those with atypical or complicated symptoms particularly when conventional pH studies have been unhelpful. A significant difficulty with impedance monitoring is that interpretation of information from these studies is dependent on a high level of expertise from the reporting physician/surgeon with a requirement for careful and time-consuming consideration of the trace, reflux episode by episode. Clear guidelines for use of impedance manometry and interpretation of results have yet to be developed, and its precise role in uncomplicated reflux remains to be clearly defined.

High-resolution manometry is a recent advance to assist the study of oesophageal function and is a more sensitive and sophisticated means of studying oesophageal function than station pull-through manometry. In high-resolution manometry, miniature pressure sensors are located every centimetre from oropharynx to stomach. Software then permits the creation of complex vector plots of oesophageal function. It appears to be of great help in defining abnormalities of oesophageal function, particularly where conventional oesophageal function studies have been unhelpful.

Impedance pH monitoring and high-resolution manometry permit highly detailed study of abnormal oesophageal function, and can generate vast quantities of clinical data, but create the, as yet unresolved, issue of how to best use this extra information to improve patient management.[6,8]

Key points 2

- Oesophageal impedance monitoring and high-resolution manometry should be considered for the investigation of patients with atypical symptoms or when conventional investigations are unhelpful or inconclusive.

PATIENT SELECTION FOR SURGERY

The aims of anti-reflux surgery are symptom control and, through this, an improvement in the overall quality of life for the patient. Appropriate selection of patients together with careful pre-operative counselling regarding symptomatic and functional outcome peri- and postoperatively are key in achieving a good outcome.

OUTCOME

MEDICAL VERSUS SURGICAL THERAPY

There are now several randomised trials comparing medical with surgical therapy for patients with reflux disease. Anti-reflux surgery has the ability to deliver a durable improved overall quality of life for patients with PPI-dependent reflux symptoms compared with standard medical therapy. Mahon et al.[9] randomised 217 patients who were treated with either optimised medical therapy or Nissen fundoplication. In this study, at 3 months and 12 months, there were significantly greater improvements in gastrointestinal and general well-being with surgery than continuing optimised medical treatment. Anvari et al.[10] randomised 104 patients with PPI-dependent reflux disease to Nissen versus continued medical treatment and also found surgery at 12 months to give better symptom control and quality-of-life scores than continued medical treatment.

The LOTUS trial is an open, parallel group, multicentre, international, randomised trial with randomisation of over 500 patients, comparing best medical therapy with Esomeprazole, against laparoscopic Nissen fundoplication. The 3-year interim analysis has found equivalence between the two treatments in control of reflux symptoms, but functional sequelae of fundoplication to be a problem within the surgical arm.[11] The REFLUX trial is a UK-based study of over 800 subjects which is designed to compare the clinical and cost-effectiveness of early laparoscopic surgery for reflux compared with standard medical therapy. This multicentre, randomised trial also has two parallel, non-randomised, preference arms and has found surgery to be more effective than medical therapy with better general and reflux-related quality-of-life outcomes up to 12 months out from surgery.[12] It is, however, expensive with estimates of £19,000 to £23,000 per quality adjusted life year (QALY), with a general threshold for cost-effectiveness set at £20,000. More severe symptoms certainly reduce the cost per QALY and may increase the possible long benefits from surgery.

Lundell et al.[13] have described long-term outcome, 7 years post-randomisation of 298 patients to either surgery or medical treatment for reflux disease. Data were available for 73%; amongst these patients, treatment success was achieved in two-thirds of surgical patients compared with 46% of medically treated subjects.

PROCEDURE SELECTION

Selection of surgical procedure remains controversial, with no consensus regarding the optimal primary procedure. We shall consider evidence regarding the important components of anti-reflux surgery separately – first, the anti-reflux procedure and, second, the hiatal repair.

Key point 3

- There is now good level 1 evidence that fundoplication is a cost-effective means of treating reflux, but functional sequelae of Nissen fundoplication can be troublesome to patients.

ANTI-REFLUX PROCEDURE

The goal of surgery for gastro-oesophageal reflux is to restore competence at the lower oesophageal sphincter. For the patient, the most important outcome is control of symptoms. Control of symptoms, however, is not always associated with improvement in lower oesophageal sphincter pressure nor with an absence of acid in the oesophagus.

Nissen fundoplication is generally considered the gold standard procedure for restoring competence at the gastro-oesophageal junction, providing a mechanical barrier to reflux. It has been studied extensively and has been found to deliver significantly raised lower oesophageal sphincter pressure, improvement in defective oesophageal peristalsis and less recurrence of erosion, stricture or ulceration in patients with erosive oesophagitis. Toupet partial posterior fundoplication involves posterior dissection and constructing a wrap over approximately two-thirds of the lower oesophageal circumference, and is more technically demanding to perform well than a Nissen fundoplication.

Several, non-randomised, case series of laparoscopic partial fundoplication have shown excellent early outcomes but an increased risk of recurrent reflux at 1 year in Toupet compared with Nissen. Fernando et al.[14] reported a non-randomised, retrospective, case series and found that those undergoing a Toupet fundoplication had a higher incidence of recurrent reflux symptoms (especially dysphagia), used more medication and were generally less satisfied with the outcome of their surgery than those patients having a Nissen fundoplication. Laws et al.[15] performed a small, randomised trial in 40 patients who were randomised to Nissen or Toupet fundoplication and found no difference between the procedures at 12 months. The 2-year follow-up of a randomised trial of 200 patients in a 2 × 2 randomised study comparing Nissen with Toupet fundoplication in patients with normal and disordered motility has now been reported.[16] Toupet and Nissen fundoplication were equally effective at managing reflux symptoms and patient satisfaction, but dysphagia following partial fundoplication was significantly less common than after Nissen(19% versus 8%). Booth et al.[17] reported 1-year follow up of a randomised trial of 127 patients randomised on the basis of pre-operative manometry to either Nissen or Toupet fundoplication. Both procedures were found to be equally effective at controlling reflux at 1 year. In both those with normal and ineffective pre-operative manometry, postoperative dysphagia (27% versus 9%) and chest pain on eating(22% versus 5%) were found to be significantly more at 1 year after Nissen compared with Toupet fundoplication. Overall, many surgeons would not yet consider there to be sufficient evidence to recommend Toupet procedure over Nissen fundoplication, largely on the basis of a higher incidence of recurrent reflux symptoms from most series. Toupet partial posterior fundoplication appears, however, to have a lower incidence of persistent dysphagia and chest pain with eating, and appears to be associated with less frequent and less severe functional symptoms. Toupet partial fundoplication is a more technical operation than the Nissen, and this may explain the apparently poor results of earlier non-randomised trials, which in turn may help to explain why it is not yet regarded as the gold standard in anti-reflux surgery.

Key point 4

- Toupet partial posterior fundoplication is as good as Nissen at controlling reflux symptoms but is associated with less dysphagia and other functional symptoms postoperatively up to 2 years.

Anterior fundoplication does not mandate a posterior dissection, although adequate intra-abdominal oesophageal length is required. Anterior fundoplication recreates the angle of His by positioning the fundus of the stomach anterior to the oesophagus and suturing this in place. Advocates of anterior fundoplication believe that it affords adequate control of reflux, whilst having significantly less functional symptoms such as dysphagia than the Nissen. Watson et al.[18] performed a randomised trial to compare anterior with Nissen fundoplication and found no important early advantages for either group in terms of reflux symptom control, and a reduction in dysphagia at 6 months in the partial fundoplication group. Although early symptom control was good following partial fundoplication, these patients had greater levels of both oesophagitis at endoscopy and acid exposure with pH monitoring. At 5 years, concerns remain about the risk of recurrent reflux[19] and these risks need to be carefully weighed against the benefits of reduced postoperative dysphagia.

Long-term outcome data from a number of trials have now started to accrue. The 10-year follow-up data in 89 of 107 patients (83%) from the Cai et al.[20] study showed no significant difference in patient-reported symptomatic outcome and overall satisfaction between anterior and Nissen fundoplication. As these data continue to accrue, they will further assist selection of the most appropriate anti-reflux procedure for patients, both in terms of optimising durable control of reflux symptoms together with minimising unwanted functional symptoms (e.g. dysphagia, chest pain, inability to belch or vomit, and early satiety).

HIATAL REPAIR

Hiatal repair with non-absorbable suture is now standard practice in all anti-reflux surgery even where there is no hiatal hernia. Failure to close the hiatus in early series contributed to very high levels of recurrent symptoms.

The management of larger hiatal defects is, however, more controversial. Simple primary suture of large defects is associated with high levels of recurrent hiatal herniation in up to 40% of patients followed by serial barium contrast radiology. It is important to note that only a small number of these patients, generally those with recurrent para-oesophageal hernia, will have persistent symptoms. In order to avoid hiatal failure, a number of approaches have been employed and these generally involve use of prosthetic material as follows.

Teflon pledgets/tape

Teflon patches are used to buttress hiatal sutures mechanically and work, in part, by means of creating a mechanical buttress and also by promoting a dense fibrotic reaction (and hence scar formation adjacent to the patch), thus rendering hiatal failure less likely in the medium- and long-term.

Prolene mesh

Prolene mesh is inexpensive and reliable in the long-term, in terms of protecting a hiatal repair. There is, however, concern among some surgeons regarding erosion of mesh through the oesophageal wall and thence into the oesophageal lumen.

PTFE mesh

Because of the lack of fibrotic reaction associated with PTFE/Goretex meshes, their use has been advocated for supporting repair of large hiatal defects. There have, however, been a number of recent reports describing erosion of this mesh through the oesophageal wall at the oesophagogastric junction including one series involving 15 cases of repair where removal of infected mesh was necessary in 3 (20%) patients.[21]

Collagen mesh

Collagen mesh has the advantage over other prosthetic materials in that it is absorbed and becomes integrated over time; as a result, it is not associated with problems related to infection or erosion. Excellent results have been reported by Lee et al.[22] using human acellular dermal matrix at 12 months in 52 patients with large hiatal hernia, as hiatal re-inforcement with recurrences was seen in only 4%. Whilst low complication rates have been reported using this technique, the long-term outcome with collagen re-inforced hiatoplasty remains unclear.

Key point 5

- Large hiatal defects have a high rate of recurrence following simple suture repair. Use of prosthetic re-inforcement reduces both the risk and extent of recurrence, but there is no clear consensus around which prosthetic should be used and when.

A variety of techniques have thus been used to re-inforce the hiatus in patients both with and without significant hiatal hernia. There is no clear, or widely accepted, guidance as to when hiatal re-inforcement should be carried out, how it should be carried out or what material should be used. It has been suggested that routine hiatal re-inforcement with prosthetic material (even in those without significant hiatal hernia) is associated with a lower incidence of hiatal failure[23] and the topic of hiatal repair seems ripe for carefully controlled, randomised study.

OESOPHAGEAL LENGTHENING PROCEDURES

The indications for oesophageal lengthening as part of an anti-reflux procedure in conjunction with hiatal repair is controversial. Whilst it is generally accepted that an adequate length of intra-abdominal oesophagus is necessary for a good outcome following fundoplication, there is no widely accepted guidance as to when lengthening is necessary and exactly how this should be done.

Laparoscopic Collis gastroplasty is advocated in those patients with a shortened oesophagus where it is not possible to obtain a satisfactory length of intra-abdominal oesophagus after oesophageal mobilisation/hiatal closure, although many question the existence of true shortened oesophagus. It is most frequently performed as a component of either para-oesophageal hernia repair or revision hiatal surgery, only rarely as part of a primary uncomplicated fundoplication, and can be technically challenging. Despite gastroplasty being performed uncommonly, meta-analysis of over 900 patients having para-oesophageal hernia repair suggests that in addition to hiatal repair technique, Collis gastroplasty by means of oesophageal lengthening may have a significant effect in terms of protecting this repair.[24]

Wedge gastroplasty has been described as an alternative means of increasing oesophageal length and early reports suggest it may be as effective as a Collis whilst being technically easier to perform.[25,26]

PARA-OESOPHAGEAL HERNIA

Para-oesophageal hernia repair can be technically difficult and, because of frequent significant co-morbidity, requires very careful clinical consideration pre-operatively. Many surgeons perform an anti-reflux procedure in combination with repair of a large hernia.

Particularly in those with significant co-morbidity, simple suture gastropexy of intrathoracic stomach to the anterior abdominal wall has been described as a quick, safe procedure that is significantly less morbid than formal hiatal repair with excision of the hernia sac, although this is unfortunately followed by a high rate of recurrent gastric herniation. Rosenberg et al.[27] described a modification of simple suture gastropexy where the hernia sac is fully dissected before gastropexy is performed and found this procedure to be safe, with recurrent hernia identified in 3 of 21 patients at 3 months, although previous data suggest that recurrence increases in frequency with time. The proposal that fundoplication is not mandatory was first described in 1998 when simple suture gastropexy suggested for incarcerated para-oesophageal hernia in the frail and elderly, although it was noted that a significant proportion of these hernias recurred early. In elective repair of large type 2 hiatal hernia (even when reflux symptoms are not present), many surgeons continue to perform a synchronous anti-reflux procedure on the basis that bulk of the wrap helps to prevent recurrent gastric herniation in to the chest. More recently, a study of 20 consecutive patients having elective repair of these hernias found that a simplified procedure with dissection and excision of the hernial sac combined with gastropexy to the anterior abdominal wall permitted excellent symptom control, making this another ideal subject for future randomised study.

DAY-CASE FUNDOPLICATION

Day-case fundoplication has been described in a number of series as feasible and safe in appropriately selected patients with high levels of patient satisfaction.[28] Complications and re-admission rates appear to be similar for day-case fundoplication to those for in-patient surgery.[29] Successful day-case fundoplication hinges around careful attention to detail, with the key factors being similar to those for laparoscopic cholecystectomy including:

1. Appropriate patient (ASA 1 or 2; body mass index < 35 kg/m^2; and social support at home).

2. Appropriate surgery (skilled surgery with operative time < 60–90 min).

3. Appropriate anaesthetic and peri-operative analgesia (pre-operative analgesia with NSAID; avoidance of morphine analgesia postoperatively; local anaesthetic infiltration of port sites; and careful avoidance of emetic agents).

> **Key points 6 and 7**
> - Anti-reflux surgery failures can be managed safely laparoscopically, with success rates similar to primary surgery.
> - Endoscopic surgery for reflux is in development. Available evidence suggests that it may improve reflux symptoms, and use of acid suppression therapy, but it does not eliminate reflux, and long-term data regarding efficacy are limited.

FAILED ANTI-REFLUX SURGERY

Whilst anti-reflux surgery produces good symptom relief in 90–95% of patients, failure occurs in 5–10% of procedures within the first 5 years. Recurrent reflux symptoms may be less severe than prior to the initial procedure and well controlled medically. For patients with significant, persistent dysphagia or recurrent reflux symptoms, re-operative surgery by means of a laparoscopic approach has been found to be feasible and safe.[30,31] Careful pre-operative work-up of patients is required with endoscopy, contrast radiology with bread/barium if dysphagia is a significant problem and pH/manometry in order to define clearly, if possible, the anatomical/mechanical cause of symptoms pre-operatively.

The principles of surgery for patients with recurrent reflux are to define the anatomical cause of failure, taking down the wrap completely, ensuring an adequate hiatal repair and reconstruction of the fundoplication. Following revision surgery for recurrent reflux, symptom control and levels of patient satisfaction are very good, being similar to that for primary surgery. For patients with dysphagia, where possible, an anatomical cause is defined and corrected. In many patients with dysphagia, however, this is not possible and in these circumstances conversion to a lesser degree of fundoplication is accompanied by improvement in dysphagia although with up to a third of patients will still experience some significant degree of dysphagia postoperatively.

Whilst very good results are achievable with revision surgery, it can be technically challenging with early series describing complication rates of up to

30%, compared with more recent series where complication rates similar to primary surgery have been achieved.

NATURAL ORIFICE SURGERY

There is currently great interest in the development of natural orifice surgery across the whole of gastrointestinal surgery. Laparoscopic anti-reflux surgery concentrates on recreating the anatomical lower-oesophageal sphincter and the following devices have been developed to perform either mucosal or full-thickness placation at the gastro-oesophageal junction.

The EndoCinch device (CR Bard; Murray Hill, NJ, USA) allows placement of a series of mucosa–mucosa plication sutures at the gastro-oesophageal junction. The device is fitted to the tip on an endoscope and suction is used to draw tissue into the device before the suture is passed through it. At 18-month follow-up, Schiefke et al.[32] reviewed 70 patients. Only 6% completely stopped PPI and 42% of sutures remained intact on endoscopic examination. In a randomised trial comparing the device with a sham procedure, Schwartz et al.[33] reported a reduced drug use in the treatment arm but no significant difference in acid exposure compared with the sham group; almost a third of patients required retreatment. Montgomery et al.[34] found improved GSRS well-being scores at 3 months but the effect was not apparent after 12 months. There were no significant changes in oesophageal acid exposure. Despite some promising short-term results, longer term outcomes appear poor and cumulative evidence suggests this treatment is not effective in reducing acid exposure.

The NDO Plicator (NDO Surgical; Mansfield, MA, USA) takes full-thickness bites performing serosa-to-serosa approximation of the stomach just distal to the gastro-oesophageal junction restoring the valve-like mechanism. The instrument is passed using a guide wire and the gastric wall is pulled into a retraction device under direct vision of the retroflexed scope before the sutures are deployed leaving a full thickness plication. The 5-year follow-up data from a multicentre cohort of outcome in 33 patients have been published.[35] In this study, two-thirds of patients with PPI-dependent reflux at the outset no longer required daily PPI. Without the benefit of randomised trials, it is not clear whether this potentially promising procedure is superior to standard medical treatment.

RADIOFREQUENCY ABLATION

The Stretta procedure (Curon Medical; Sunnyvale, CA, USA) is a controlled delivery of radiofrequency (RF) energy via an inflatable endoscopically placed balloon-basket containing four penetrating needle electrodes. The tips of these electrodes deliver energy at multiple locations in the distal oesophagus and gastric cardia whilst the temperature is controlled by thermocouples at the base and tip of each needle together with irrigation of sterile water. A study[36] of over 500 patients suggested that 77% of patients showed improvement of symptoms and this effect persisted for over 12 months. A randomised, sham-controlled study[37] of 64 patients confirmed improvement in health-related quality-of-life scores at both 6 months and 12 months; however, there were no statistically significant differences between PPI use and distal acid exposure times. Limited, longer term data are available and these suggest that the Stretta offers improvement in reflux symptoms, with reduction in PPI usage, but do not render patients symptom-free.[38]

INJECTABLES

The aim of injectable treatments for GORD is to add bulk to the oesophagus at the gastro-oesophageal junction, in order to augment a poorly functioning lower oesophageal sphincter.

The Gatekeeper system (Medtronic; Minneapolis, MN, USA) involves the injection of 3–6 polyacrylonitrile-based hydrogel rods into the submucosa of the oesophagus. These take on water and enlarge, reducing reflux. In a small group of patients, Cicala reported improvement in GORD health-related quality-of-life scores after 6 months. Fockens et al.[39] showed significant reduction in lower oesophageal acid exposure together with increased LOSP in a study of 67 patients. Over 70% of the implants were retained at 6 months. There were two complications with one pharyngeal perforation.

Enteryx (Boston Scientific; Natick, MA, USA), an injectable solution of 8% ethylene vinyl alcohol, has also been developed for submucosal injection. A circumferential injection tightens the gastro-oesophageal junction. A sham-controlled trial of 64 patients showed a significant reduction in both PPI usage and on-going need for PPI at 6 months following injection.[40] Safety concerns were raised following two deaths, one of which involved injection of Enteryx into the aorta, and pneumomediastinum in a further patient.

Because of patient safety concerns, the above two injectable systems have now been withdrawn.

PHARMACOTHERAPY

This can currently deliver symptomatic relief by altering the composition of oesophageal refluxate with proton pump inhibitors or improving gastric emptying with prokinetic agents. The most attractive pharmacological approach to management of reflux disease lies with the development of an agent that modulates activity of the lower oesophageal sphincter and, therefore, controls gastro-oesophageal reflux, with little or no disturbance to other aspects of oesophageal motor function. An animal study has shown Baclofen (a GABA type B receptor agonist) dose dependently inhibits transient lower oesophageal sphincter relaxations in dogs, although it is not yet clear whether this can be translated into a clinically useful effect in humans.

Key points for clinical practice

- Reflux disease is increasing in prevalence, together with oesophageal adenocarcinoma and this may mediated by increasing levels of obesity.

- Oesophageal impedance monitoring and high-resolution manometry should be considered for the investigation of patients with atypical symptoms or when conventional investigations are unhelpful or inconclusive.

Key points for clinical practice (*continued*)

- There is now good level 1 evidence that fundoplication is a cost-effective means of treating reflux, but functional sequelae of Nissen fundoplication can be troublesome to patients.

- Toupet partial posterior fundoplication is as good as Nissen at controlling reflux symptoms but is associated with less dysphagia and other functional symptoms postoperatively up to 2 years.

- Large hiatal defects have a high rate of recurrence following simple suture repair. Use of prosthetic re-inforcement reduces both the risk and extent of recurrence, but there is no clear consensus around which prosthetic should be used and when.

- Anti-reflux surgery failures can be managed safely laparoscopically, with success rates similar to primary surgery.

- Endoscopic surgery for reflux is in development. Available evidence suggests that it may improve reflux symptoms, and use of acid suppression therapy, but it does not eliminate reflux, and long-term data regarding efficacy are limited.

References

1. Loffeld RJ. van der Putten AB. Rising incidence of reflux oesophagitis in patients undergoing upper gastrointestinal endoscopy. *Digestion* 2003; **68**: 141–144.
2. Nandurkar S, Locke 3rd GR, Fett S, Zinsmeister AR, Cameron AJ, Talley NJ. Relationship between body mass index, diet, exercise and gastro-oesophageal reflux symptoms in a community. *Aliment Pharmacol Ther* 2004; **20**: 497–505.
3. Pandolfino JE, Zhang QG, Ghosh SK, Han A, Boniquit C, Kahrilas PJ. Transient lower esophageal sphincter relaxations and reflux: mechanistic analysis using concurrent fluoroscopy and high-resolution manometry. *Gastroenterology* 2006; **131**: 1725–1733.
4. Wu JC, Mui LM, Cheung CM, Chan Y, Sung JJ. Obesity is associated with increased transient lower esophageal sphincter relaxation. *Gastroenterology* 2007; **132**: 883–889.
5. Lagergren J, Bergström R, Lindgren A, Nyrén O. Symptomatic gastroesophageal reflux as a risk factor for esophageal adenocarcinoma. *N Engl J Med* 1999; **340**: 825–831.
6. Bredenoord AJ, Smout AJ. Esophageal motility testing: impedance-based transit measurement and high-resolution manometry. *Gastroenterol Clin North Am* 2008; **37**: 775–791.
7. del Genio G, Tolone S, del Genio F *et al*. Prospective assessment of patient selection for antireflux surgery by combined multichannel intraluminal impedance pH monitoring. *J Gastrointest Surg* 2008; **12**: 1491–1496.
8. Kahrilas PJ, Sifrim D. High-resolution manometry and impedance-pH/manometry: valuable tools in clinical and investigational esophagology. *Gastroenterology* 2008; **135**: 756–769.
9. Mahon D, Rhodes M, Decadt B *et al*. Randomized clinical trial of laparoscopic Nissen fundoplication compared with proton-pump inhibitors for treatment of chronic gastro-oesophageal reflux. *Br J Surg* 2005; **92**: 695–699.
10. Anvari M, Allen C, Marshall J *et al*. A randomized controlled trial of laparoscopic Nissen fundoplication versus proton pump inhibitors for treatment of patients with chronic gastroesophageal reflux disease: one-year follow-up. *Surg Innov* 2006; **13**: 238–249.
11. Lundell L, Attwood S, Ell C *et al*.; LOTUS Trial Collaborators. Comparing laparoscopic antireflux surgery with Esomeprazole in the management of patients with chronic gastro-oesophageal reflux disease: a 3-year interim analysis of the LOTUS trial. *Gut* 2008; **57**: 1207–1213.

12. Grant A, Wileman S, Ramsay C *et al.*; REFLUX Trial Group. The effectiveness and cost-effectiveness of minimal access surgery amongst people with gastro-oesophageal reflux disease – a UK collaborative study. The REFLUX trial. *Health Technol Assess* 2008; **12**: 1–181.

13. Lundell L, Miettinen P, Myrvold HE *et al.*; Nordic GORD Study Group. Seven-year follow-up of a randomized clinical trial comparing proton-pump inhibition with surgical therapy for reflux oesophagitis. *Br J Surg* 2007; **94**: 198–203.

14. Fernando HC, Luketich JD, Christie NA, Ikramuddin S, Schauer PR. Outcomes of laparoscopic Toupet compared to laparoscopic Nissen fundoplication. *Surg Endosc* 2002; **16**: 905–908.

15. Laws HL, Clements RH, Swillie CM. A randomized, prospective comparison of the Nissen fundoplication versus the Toupet fundoplication for gastroesophageal reflux disease. *Ann Surg* 1997; **225**: 647–653.

16. Strate U, Emmermann A, Fibbe C, Layer P, Zornig C. Laparoscopic fundoplication: Nissen versus Toupet two-year outcome of a prospective randomized study of 200 patients regarding preoperative esophageal motility. *Surg Endosc* 2008; **22**: 21–30.

17. Booth MI, Stratford J, Jones L, Dehn TC. Randomized clinical trial of laparoscopic total (Nissen) versus posterior partial (Toupet) fundoplication for gastro-oesophageal reflux disease based on preoperative oesophageal manometry. *Br J Surg* 2008; **95**: 57–63.

18. Watson DI, Jamieson GG, Pike GK, Davies N, Richardson M, Devitt PG. Prospective randomized double-blind trial between laparoscopic Nissen fundoplication and anterior partial fundoplication. *Br J Surg* 1999; **86**: 123–130.

19. Ludemann R, Watson DI, Jamieson GG, Game PA, Devitt PG. Five-year follow-up of a randomized clinical trial of laparoscopic total versus anterior 180 degrees fundoplication. *Br J Surg* 2005; **92**: 240–243.

20. Cai W, Watson DI, Lally CJ, Devitt PG, Game PA, Jamieson GG. Ten-year clinical outcome of a prospective randomized clinical trial of laparoscopic Nissen versus anterior 180 (degrees) partial fundoplication. *Br J Surg* 2008; **95**: 1501–1505.

21. Griffith PS, Valenti V, Qurashi K, Martinez-Isla A Rejection of Goretex mesh used in prosthetic cruroplasty: a case series. *Int J Surg* 2008; **6**: 106–109.

22. Lee YK, James E, Bochkarev V, Vitamvas M, Oleynikov D. Long-term outcome of cruroplasty reinforcement with human acellular dermal matrix in large paraesophageal hiatal hernia. *J Gastrointest Surg* 2008; **12**: 811–815.

23. Johnson JM, Carbonell AM, Carmody BJ *et al.* Laparoscopic mesh hiatoplasty for paraesophageal hernias and fundoplications: a critical analysis of the available literature. *Surg Endosc* 2006; **20**: 362–366.

24. Rathore MA, Andrabi SI, Bhatti MI, Najfi SM, McMurray A. Metanalysis of recurrence after laparoscopic repair of paraesophageal hernia. *J Soc Laparosc Surg* 2007; **11**: 456–460.

25. Terry ML, Vernon A, Hunter JG. Stapled-wedge Collis gastroplasty for the shortened esophagus. *Am J Surg* 2004; **188**: 195–199.

26. Whitson BA, Hoang CD, Boettcher AK, Dahlberg PS, Andrade RS, Maddaus MA. Wedge gastroplasty and reinforced crural repair: important components of laparoscopic giant or recurrent hiatal hernia repair. *J Thorac Cardiovasc Surg* 2006; **132**: 1196–1202.

27. Rosenberg J, Jacobsen B, Fischer A. Fast-track giant paraoesophageal hernia repair using a simplified laparoscopic technique. *Langenbecks Arch Surg* 2006; **391**: 38–42.

28. Triboulet JP. The safety of the same-day discharge for selected patients after laparoscopic fundoplication: a prospective cohort study. *Am J Surg* 2007; **194**: 279–282.

29. Ng R, Mullin EJ, Maddern GJ. Systematic review of day-case laparoscopic Nissen fundoplication. *Aust NZ J Surg* 2005; **75**: 160–164.

30. Khajanchee YS, O'Rourke R, Cassera MA, Gatta P, Hansen PD, Swanström LL. Laparoscopic reintervention for failed antireflux surgery: subjective and objective outcomes in 176 consecutive patients. *Arch Surg* 2007; **142**: 785–901.

31. Byrne JP, Smithers BM, Nathanson LK, Martin I, Ong HS, Gotley DC. Outcome after re-operation for failed anti reflux surgery. *Br J Surg* 2005; **92**: 996–1001.

32. Schiefke I, Zabel-Langhennig A, Neumann S, Feisthammel J, Moessner J, Caca K. Long term failure of endoscopic gastroplication (EndoCinch). *Gut* 2005; **54**: 752–758.

33. Schwartz MP, Wellink H, Gooszen HG, Conchillo JM, Samsom M, Smout AJ. Endoscopic gastroplication for the treatment of gastro-oesophageal reflux disease: a randomised,

sham-controlled trial. *Gut* 2007; **56**: 20–28.

34. Montgomery M, Håkanson B, Ljungqvist O, Ahlman B, Thorell A. Twelve months' follow-up after treatment with the EndoCinch endoscopic technique for gastro-oesophageal reflux disease: a randomized, placebo-controlled study. *Scand J Gastroenterol* 2006; **41**: 1382–1389.

35. Pleskow D, Rothstein R, Kozarek R *et al*. Endoscopic full-thickness plication for the treatment of GERD: Five-year long-term multicenter results. *Surg Endosc* 2008; **22**: 326–332.

36. Wolfsen HC, Richards WO. The Stretta procedure for the treatment of GERD: a registry of 558 patients. *J Laparoendosc Adv Surg Tech A* 2002; **12**: 395–402.

37. Triadafilopoulos G, DiBaise JK, Nostrant TT *et al*. The Stretta procedure for the treatment of GERD: 6 and 12 month follow-up of the U.S. open label trial. *Gastrointest Endosc* 2002; **55**: 149–156.

38. Noar MD, Lotfi-Emran S. Sustained improvement in symptoms of GERD and antisecretory drug use: 4-year follow-up of the Stretta procedure. *Gastrointest Endosc* 2007; **65**: 367–372.

39. Fockens P, Bruno MJ, Gabbrielli A *et al*. Endoscopic augmentation of the lower esophageal sphincter for the treatment of gastroesophageal reflux disease: multicenter study of the Gatekeeper reflux repair system. *Endoscopy* 2004; **36**: 682–689.

40. Devière J, Costamagna G, Neuhaus H *et al*. Nonresorbable copolymer implantation for gastroesophageal reflux disease: a randomized sham-controlled multicenter trial. *Gastroenterology* 2005; **128**: 532–540.

Bawantha Gamage Tan Arulampalam

11

Recent advances in laparoscopic surgery

Laparoscopic surgery has developed beyond recognition in the last two decades. The momentum for this surgical revolution came in the mid-1980s, particularly after the first laparoscopic cholecystectomy performed by Mouret in 1987. The aim of this chapter is to address recent innovations in technology and instrumentation as well as developments in the various subspecialities of general surgery. The reader should also gain an insight into future developments including robotic surgery and Natural Orifice Transluminal Endoscopic Surgery (NOTES).

INSTRUMENTATION

The ability to view structures within a body cavity in perfect two-dimensional, high-definition clarity on flat screens is a practical reality today. The advances in optics since the first Hopkins scopes has been astonishing. Three chip cameras coupled with high quality laparoscopes mean that it is possible to tackle most pathologies within the peritoneal cavity. The surgeon can make use of 30° and 45° laparoscopes in order to view structures within narrow confines and where access has previously been difficult.

Once these basic requirements have been met, important refinements were introduced into the operating theatre environment. The use of gravity as a retractor meant that it is now essential to operate with the patient on a table that can be moved with complete freedom in all three axes intra-operatively. Consequently, techniques of securing the patient reliably on the table without causing obstruction to the surgeon or anaesthetist, neurovascular damage or

Bawantha Gamage MS MRCS
Laparoscopic Fellow, The ICENI Centre, Colchester General Hospital, Turner Road, Colchester, Essex CO4 5JL, UK

Tan Arulampalam MD FRCS (for correspondence)
Consultant Laparoscopic Surgeon and Service Director, The ICENI Centre, Colchester General Hospital, Turner Road, Colchester, Essex CO4 5JL, UK. E-mail: tan.arulampalam@colchesterhospital.nhs.uk

skin trauma have been developed. These range from simple straps and supports to sophisticated gel pads and beanbags. Another key development has been the integrated laparoscopic operating theatre, with all screens and essential equipment suspended on ceiling-mounted pendants with command and control units housed peripherally in the theatre. This means that there is far less movement of equipment between theatre suites and, consequently, reduced damage to equipment and those that move them. The ability to perform multiquadrant surgery and move monitors rather than complete stack systems reduces stress during the operation and time taken for procedures.

The instrumentation used to perform the procedures should be classified in two groups: (i) the energy units for cutting and coagulation; and (ii) the endomechanical instruments such as ports, graspers and various retracting devices. Developments in energy platforms have been particularly encouraging with the introduction of safe equipment for cutting and coagulating tissue. Dissectors such as those developed by Ethicon Endosurgery (Harmonic™; Fig 1), Lotus and Olympus Keymed (Sonosurg™) work using the principles of ultrasonic energy to cause tissue coagulation. More conventional bipolar diathermy dissectors, shears and probes use heat energy from an alternating current. The Ligasure™ device is a sophisticated tool for delivering this energy through a hand piece that crushes tissue, coagulates and, at the appropriate time, the surgeon pulls the trigger for an integrated knife to divide the tissues within the jaws. All these instruments become hot during use; therefore, if tissues are unintentionally touched or handled, the likelihood of damage is present.[1] Both the Harmonic™ and Ligasure™ are certainly available as 5-mm instruments and both can coagulate and seal vessels of 5-mm and 7-mm calibre if used according to the manufacturers' guidelines.

Equally important has been the development in endomechanical devices. These fall into five broad categories: trocars and ports, grasping and retracting devices, prosthetic materials, procedural instruments and, finally, endoscopic stapling devices.

The arguments for trocars being re-usable or single-use present two counterpoints which have to be resolved at a local level depending on the resources and expertise available, volume of procedures and, of course, consideration for sterilisation services. A reliable supply and concerns in some quarters with regards theoretical risks of infection mean there is a strong case to reconsider conventional wisdom. An important final point to mention at this stage is the role of hand-assist or hand-port devices, designed so that the surgeon can insert their hand into the peritoneal cavity through a plastic stoma, re-establish a pneumoperitoneum by closing an iris-like portion of the

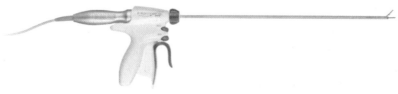

Fig. 1 The Harmonic ACE™ shears which use ultrasonic energy to cut, coagulate and dissect.

hand port and, thereby, maintain a seal. These devices allow the surgeon, particularly those in the early stages of their learning curve, to acquire laparoscopic skills when performing advanced procedures. The cost of the device has to be balanced against time saved, if any. There may be a tendency to lose some of the benefits of a pure laparoscopic dissection such as smaller wounds and good visualisation. The uptake of hand-port devices is relatively low, however.

Various endomechanical retractors are available for the broad spectrum of general surgical procedures. It is advisable that, when undergoing training for laparoscopic surgery, particular emphasis is placed by the trainee on the very specific modular nature of a laparoscopic operation and becoming familiar with the necessary equipment.

Prosthesis technology has made great strides with a variety of strong, durable and well-handling meshes available for hernia repair. These can be delivered easily and fixed with reliability. This along with training has seen a large increase in surgeons taking on the laparoscopic approach for hernia repair. The introduction of dual or composite meshes (*i.e.* a prosthetic material coated on the underside with a biological material) should, in theory, reduce intraperitoneal adhesions and small bowel fistulation.[2]

Endoscopic stapling technology is extremely sophisticated with manufacturers able to provide devices suitable for most procedures that require stapling along with transection of tissue, whether this be a gastrointestinal mucosal viscus or vascular structures. If the stapler is to be used in the pelvis or around the hiatus, additional consideration should be given to access and point at which the instrument articulates. Of particular concern is the use of articulating staplers in the fixed, bony pelvis where an angled staple line can lead to multiple firing of the stapler and a theoretical risk of ischaemia to parts of the staple line. Staplers can vary greatly in terms of firing mechanisms and feedback signals that indicate successful use as well as the distance that the jaws open, length of the staple line and point at which they articulate. Of great importance is the number of rows of staples and the height of the staples.

Key points 1–3

TECHNOLOGY ADVANCES

- Major progress has been made in terms of operating room environment including the availability and affordability of integrated operating systems, high quality optics and operating tables.

- Key improvements in the instrumentation available has made virtually any procedure possible within the abdominal cavity. These include the development of the novel energy platforms for cutting, coagulating and dissecting as well as endomechanical devices for stapling, transecting and anastomosing.

- A working knowledge of all the hardware and instrumentation available facilitates competencies and accelerated learning up the learning curve.

COLORECTAL SURGERY

Laparoscopic colorectal surgery has been given fresh impetus with the recent publication of large-scale, multi-centre, randomised controlled trials (RCTs) conducted world-wide. Laparoscopic colorectal surgery is technically challenging due to the nature of the organ, necessitating surgery in multiple abdominal quadrants. As well as the technical aspects of the surgery, there were significant concerns with regards the oncological safety of the technique, in particular the issue of local recurrence in rectal cancer surgery and port site recurrence. There have been large-scale studies, incorporated into the meta-analysis by Abrahams and colleagues,[3] that have shown the short-term benefits of less postoperative pain, better cosmesis, faster recovery of gastrointestinal function and reduced cardiorespiratory complications.

These findings were elegantly demonstrated in the single-centre, randomised, controlled study by Lacy et al.,[4] published in *The Lancet*. The multicentre RCTs have all matured; of particular interest are the COST study from the US,[5] the UK MRC CLASICC study[6] and the COLOR study from Europe.[7] COST and COLOR both looked at colon cancer surgery, whereas CLASICC included patients with rectal cancer. These trials demonstrated no difference in overall survival or, indeed, any difference in oncological outcome. Surgeons were selected for CLASICC and COST if they had performed a minimum of 20 cases. This is early in the learning curve as demonstrated in CLASICC where year 1 conversion rates were 38% compared with 16% in year 6. The concerns about rectal cancer surgery remain and this relates now more to the technical challenge and the available instrumentation to work within the confines of the pelvis. Instrumentation, particularly graspers for the rectum, is in constant development, while others are advocating the use of robotics to tackle the problem. The initial concerns raised in the CLASICC trial with regards the slightly increased involvement of circumferential resection margins in the laparoscopic group has not translated into an increased local recurrence rate.

The safety and feasibility have, therefore, been satisfactorily demonstrated and the UK National Institute for Health and Clinical Excellence (NICE) appraisal has examined this technique.[8] The UK Department of Health has sanctioned funding of a national laparoscopic colorectal training programme in England with plans for a Welsh programme also proposed. This programme involves initially up to 8 centres which have tendered various models of training for consultant surgeons based on the 'trainee' performing in the region of 20 cases under supervision. The success of this programme will be hard to gauge for a few years, but the intention to provide high-quality training for surgeons in the hope of avoiding major procedure-related morbidity and mortality has to be commended.

Surgery for inflammatory bowel disease is currently feasible and successful, especially for conditions such as Crohn's disease where the likelihood of repeat surgery is high and the opportunity to avoid intra-abdominal adhesions is of great benefit. Surgery for acute colitis requires adequate operating facilities and a surgeon with substantial experience due to the nature of the technical challenge. Diverticular disease and its complications also lend themselves to the laparoscopic approach; however, it should be noted that the technical demands are high and the chances of conversion to open surgery are greater than with malignancy as a general rule.[9]

UPPER GASTROINTESTINAL SURGERY

There has been great change in the field of minimally invasive oesophagectomy (MIO) and surgery for metabolic disease and obesity. Fundoplication for gastrointestinal reflux disease (GORD) is now the standard of care for surgical treatment for this condition. Although cholecystectomy is now a core laparoscopic operation, synchronous common bile duct exploration (CBDE) has not been widely adopted. This is due to the wide-spread availability of ERCP coupled with the relative lack of equipment for CBDE and appropriate surgical training.

Oesophagectomy is associated with relatively high morbidity and mortality. Trauma of access and postoperative pain have a significant impact on outcome. The minimally invasive approach has several advantages including less pain, less trauma and better access to the thorax and abdomen. The work of Berrisford and colleagues[10] confirmed the excellent earlier results published by Luketich and co-workers demonstrating that MIO can be performed safely with low morbidity and morality. The series of Berrisford *et al.*[10] is the largest published in the UK with 70 out of 77 patients in an unselected group undergoing MIO with a mortality of only 1%, morbidity of 47% and mean overall and disease-free survival of 35 months and 33 months, respectively. The key aspect of this procedure is the adequacy of training and auditing outcomes by means of meticulous data collection.

There were 8000 bariatric procedures performed for weight loss in the UK last year, a number that will increase dramatically in the coming years. In 2006, bariatric procedure overtook cholecystectomy as the commonest major general surgical operation in the US. NICE approval was given for weight-loss surgery as long ago as 2002, but uptake has been evidently slow. The importance of a working knowledge of the operations has been voiced by the Association of Laparoscopic Surgeons of Great Britain and Ireland (ALSGBI). As most procedures tend to be performed in private hospitals and the surgery lends itself to early discharge within 48 h, patients who suffer complications naturally present at local NHS emergency departments. Prompt clinical assessment with appropriate imaging, whether simple contrast studies or computed tomography (CT), and early communication with the original operating surgeon with intervention, if necessary, are more likely to lead to favourable outcomes. Laparoscopic gastric banding was introduced in the UK in 1997. These may slip, tighten or erode. Roux-en-Y gastric bypass and biliopancreatic bypass may be associated with stenosis of the gastro-jejunostomy, haemorrhage or intestinal obstruction. In addition, one has to be mindful of nutritional deficiencies particularly with sleeve gastrectomy and vertical band gastroplasty.

There are around one billion people world-wide who are overweight. With obesity come complications, including ischaemic heart disease, musculo-skeletal problems, psychological illnesses and metabolic disease. The latter is of interest as type II diabetes can be cured surgically in a majority of patients even before any evidence of weight loss.[11] The mechanisms are not entirely clear but it is proposed that calorie restriction, various changes in gastrointestinal hormones and the fat content of adipocytes play an important role. Cohen and colleagues[12] elegantly demonstrated reduction in HbA1c without significant weight loss in non-obese patients who underwent duodenojejunal bypass. The Endobarrier, endoscopically deployed in the duodenum in order to simulate a similar bypass, resulted in improvements in diabetes.[13]

VASCULAR SURGERY

The appeal of minimally invasive techniques for aortic surgery stems from the possibility of reducing postoperative pain and stress. Although there has been keen interest and uptake in endovascular techniques, the evidence for laparoscopic aortic surgery has been slower in maturing. The indications for laparoscopic aortic surgery include abdominal aortic aneurysms, aortoiliac occlusive disease and mesenteric revascularisation. The repair of endoleaks following endovascular aortic stenting and more recently the removal of unsalvagable endovascular shunt-grafts. It is feasible to approach the aorta directly (transperitoneal) having repositioned the bowel; however, the most favoured method involves a lateral (retroperitoneal) approach with the initial step being to mobilise the colon and approach the aorta from the left side.

The operative times are longer for laparoscopic operations in three non-randomised, controlled trials.[14–16] One non-randomised study has compared endovascular stenting with laparoscopic repair; although there was a trend to increased operating time with the former, a statistically significant difference in time was not shown.[17] Lengths of stay were reduced with laparoscopic repair but were similar following stenting. The mortality varied between 3% and 10% with a rate of complications varying between less than 1% and 4%. Overall, the initial results are impressive, but the technique is still maturing and more outcome data, particularly for the few centres in the UK, are awaited.

ENDOCRINE, HEPATOPANCREATIC AND TRANSPLANT SURGERY

The laparoscopic approach to the adrenal gland has become increasingly favoured by surgeons and patients alike for the reasons of decreased pain, shorter hospital stay, and improved cosmesis. Liver metastases can safely be tackled using a laparoscopic approach especially with the availability of a variety of methods of haemostasis such as CUSA, Harmonic, Ligasure and staplers. Outcomes are good and short-term benefits make the approach attractive to patients. Finally, one has to note that minimally invasive techniques for transplantation are now feasible.

HERNIA SURGERY

There are well over 100,000 groin hernia repairs carried out in the UK per year and the impact of laparoscopic repair has been profound. Laparoscopic repair is associated with less chronic postoperative pain, earlier return to work and lower incidence of wound infection.[18] The major question now is which is the best approach – the transabdominal preperitoneal (TAPP) or the totally extraperitoneal approach (TEPP). Both have a low rate of recurrence but early reports of TAPP were associated with complications, which have largely been overcome. TEPP is the harder technique to learn but there is a significant body of literature favouring this over TAPP.

Incisional hernias are a significant general surgical problem. Published data suggest that the laparoscopic approach is associated with low recurrence rates, less pain and shorter hospital stays. Recurrence may be reduced in laparoscopic series due to the accurate identification of all defects and placement of a sufficiently large mesh across all these defects.[19]

EMERGENCY SURGERY

The field of emergency surgery is set to alter significantly over the coming years with changes in junior surgeons' working patterns and an even greater emphasis on quality of care. Surgeons and their teams are increasingly adopting a system where they may be on-call for several consecutive days and give up all elective commitments. This, alongside the provision of dedicated emergency theatres, means that supervised training in laparoscopic surgery for appendicitis, cholecystitis, perforated peptic ulcer disease, diverticulitis and even small bowel obstruction can be undertaken. A recent Cochrane review has recommended laparoscopic appendicectomy confirming the impression that this procedure is associated with shorter hospital stay after surgery, reduced pain and wound infections.[20]

Similarly, the ability to perform laparoscopic repair of perforated duodenal ulcers gives patients great benefit, particularly by avoiding a painful upper abdominal scar, which can compromise breathing. Laparoscopic cholecystectomy performed as an emergency is more wide-spread and the ability to deal with difficult anatomy and disease by performing a subtotal resection has improved safety.[21] The other areas where the laparoscopic approach has altered conventional attitudes is subtotal colectomy for acute colitis and laparoscopy for diverticulitis and small bowel obstruction. However, operating time is generally longer and the surgical expertise required greater.

Finally, emergency surgical mortality due to large bowel obstruction carries a significant mortality and morbidity. The ability to decompress the bowel using colonic stents and then offer patients the opportunity of an urgent laparoscopic resection may have huge implications for this field.

PAEDIATRICS

As with all areas of general surgery, paediatric surgery has realised enormous benefits from the laparoscopic revolution. It is possible to perform a wide range of procedures; however, the cautions associated with performing surgery on children apply to laparoscopic surgery. These include adequate training, appropriate case selection and sufficient back up in the event of complications. In addition, one must be aware that fetal surgery is a growing field in its own right. This chapter does not address paediatric laparoscopy in detail, although Losty's excellent review offers more detail.[22]

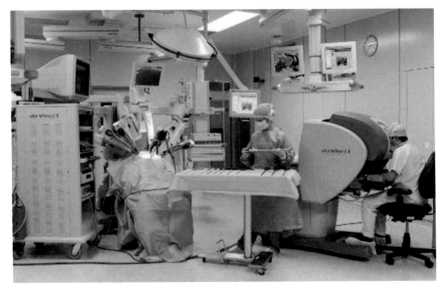

Fig. 2 The Da Vinci™ robot in clinical use with the surgeon remote from the site of surgery.

THE FUTURE

The role of robotics (Fig. 2) in laparoscopic surgery is one that has caused much debate although acceptance in the field of urology is unparalleled.[23] The cost of a fixed system including maintenance means these devices are not widely available. Their role in certain procedures such as rectal surgery and assistance in oesophageal surgery can be strongly argued; however, the current systems offer limited capability. Degrees of freedom of each instrument enable precise dissection and, coupled with adequate access, allow for excellent visceral mobilisation. The future for robotics in general surgery may, however, be linked to the rapidly developing field of NOTES and associated technology. Robotics coupled with flexible endoscopes and laparoscopes may offer versatile instruments better able to deal with the limitations of the pneumoperitoneal environment.

NOTES is currently considered an area of clinical research with animal models for cholecystectomy amongst other procedures. World-wide, there has been an explosion in interest and a substantial number of human NOTES procedures carried out. Close examination is required as to the nature of the procedures, the methodology and the outcome data. As yet, the advantages have not been unequivocally demonstrated and a degree of regulation by organisations such as Natural Orifice Surgery Consortium for Assessment and Research (NOSCARS) has proved an effective way ensuring close peer review and collaboration.[24] The ALSGBI has published guidance for NOTES development,[25] which echo many of the guiding principles behind NOSCARS.

CONCLUSIONS

The field of laparoscopic surgery has rapidly evolved, but there are many areas outlined in this chapter that require significant surgeon training, financial and human resources as well as supporting infrastructure. The main advances have been technological, which in turn have led to new procedures being developed or minimally invasive principles being applied to conventional open surgery. It is essential that two areas are noted when considering this subject; first, the training required and how this is delivered. Second, one must consider the resources available. The field is constantly in flux with the advent of robotics and NOTES. Both these areas need to be kept in mind when assessing the future of laparoscopic general surgery.

Key points for clinical practice

TECHNOLOGY ADVANCES

- Major progress has been made in terms of operating room environment including the availability and affordability of integrated operating systems, high quality optics and operating tables.

- Key improvements in the instrumentation available has made virtually any procedure possible within the abdominal cavity. These include the development of the novel energy platforms for cutting, coagulating and dissecting as well as endomechanical devices for stapling, transecting and anastomosing.

- A working knowledge of all the hardware and instrumentation available facilitates competencies and accelerated learning up the learning curve.

FUTURE HORIZONS

- Areas of great progress other than the technical issues include establishment of competency-based training programmes and direct observation of procedures.

- Future developments, which will certainly impact on every surgeon, include the development of robotic technology close to the patient, flexible laparoscopy and NOTES.

- Pioneering surgeons and trainees need to be aware of current guidelines, ethical issues and clinical governance when undertaking new procedures.

References

1. Huscher CG, Lirici MM, Anastasi A, Sansonetti A, Amini M. Laparoscopic cholecystectomy by harmonic dissection. *Surg Endosc* 1999; **13**: 1256–1257.
2. Duffy AJ, Hogle NJ, LaPerle KM, Fowler DL. Comparison of two composite meshes using two fixation devices in a porcine laparoscopic ventral hernia repair model. *Hernia* 2004; **8**: 358–364.
3. Abraham NS, Byrne CM, Young JM, Solomon MJ. Meta-analysis of non-randomized comparative studies of the short-term outcomes of laparoscopic resection for colorectal cancer. *Aust NZ J Surg* 2007; **77**: 508–516.
4. Lacy AM, Garcia-Valdecasas JC, Delgado S *et al.* Laparoscopy-assisted colectomy versus open colectomy for treatment of non-metastatic colon cancer: a randomised trial. *Lancet*

2002; **359**: 2224–2229.

5. Fleshman J, Sargent DJ, Green E *et al*. Laparoscopic colectomy for cancer is not inferior to open surgery based on 5-year data from the COST Study Group trial. *Ann Surg* 2007; **246**: 655–662.

6. Jayne DG, Guillou PJ, Thorpe H *et al*. Randomized trial of laparoscopic-assisted resection of colorectal carcinoma: 3-year results of the UK MRC CLASICC Trial Group. *J Clin Oncol* 2007; **25**: 3061–3068.

7. Veldkamp R, Kuhry E, Hop WC *et al*. Laparoscopic surgery versus open surgery for colon cancer: short-term outcomes of a randomised trial. *Lancet Oncol* 2005; **6**: 477–484.

8. The National Institute for Health and Clinical Excellence. *Colorectal Cancer – Laparoscopic Surgery*. London: NICE, 2006 <www.nice.org.uk/80/guidance/index.jsp?action=byID&r=true&o=11588>.

9. Engledow AH, Pakzad F, Ward NJ, Arulampalam T, Motson RW. Laparoscopic resection of diverticular fistulae: a 10-year experience. *Colorectal Dis* 2007; **9**: 632–634.

10. Berrisford RG, Wajed SA, Sanders D, Rucklidge MW. Short-term outcomes following total minimally invasive oesophagectomy. *Br J Surg* 2008; **95**: 602–610.

11. Greve JW, Rubino F. Bariatric surgery for metabolic disorders. *Br J Surg* 2008; **95**: 1313–1314.

12. Cohen RV, Schiavon CA, Pinheiro JS, Correa JL, Rubino F. Duodenal-jejunal bypass for the treatment of type 2 diabetes in patients with body mass index of 22–34 kg/m^2: a report of 2 cases. *Surg Obes Relat Dis* 2007; **3**: 195–197.

13. Rodriguez-Grunert L, Galvao Neto MP, Alamo M, Ramos AC, Baez PB, Tarnoff M. First human experience with endoscopically delivered and retrieved duodenal–jejunal bypass sleeve. *Surg Obes Relat Dis* 2008; **4**: 55–59.

14. Kolvenbach R. Hand-assisted laparoscopic abdominal aortic aneurysm repair. *Semin Laparosc Surg* 2001; **8**: 168–177.

15. Edoga JK, Asgarian K, Singh D *et al*. Laparoscopic surgery for abdominal aortic aneurysms. Technical elements of the procedure and a preliminary report of the first 22 patients. *Surg Endosc* 1998; **12**: 1064–1072.

16. Castronuovo Jr JJ, James KV, Resnikoff M, McLean ER, Edoga JK. Laparoscopic-assisted abdominal aortic aneurysmectomy. *J Vasc Surg* 2000; **32**: 224–233.

17. Kolvenbach R, Ceshire N, Pinter L, Da Silva L, Deling O, Kasper AS. Laparoscopy-assisted aneurysm resection as a minimal invasive alternative in patients unsuitable for endovascular surgery. *J Vasc Surg* 2001; **34**: 216–221.

18. Motson RW. Why does NICE not recommend laparoscopic herniorraphy? *BMJ* 2002; **324**: 1092–1094.

19. Motson RW, Engledow AH, Medhurst C, Adib R, Warren SJ. Laparoscopic incisional hernia repair with a self-centring suture. *Br J Surg* 2006; **93**: 1549–1553.

20. Sauerland S, Lefering R, Neugebauer EA. Laparoscopic versus open surgery for suspected appendicitis. *Cochrane Database Syst Rev* 2004; (4): CD001546.

21. Philips JA, Lawes DA, Cook AJ *et al*. The use of laparoscopic subtotal cholecystectomy for complicated cholelithiasis. *Surg Endosc* 2008; **22**: 1697–1700.

22. Losty PD. Recent advances: paediatric surgery. *BMJ* 1999; **318**: 1668–1672.

23. Bastide C, Paparel P, Guillonneau B. Minimally invasive surgery in oncologic urology: a recent review. *Curr Opin Urol* 2008; **18**: 190–197.

24. Rattner D, Kalloo A. ASGE/SAGES Working Group on Natural Orifice Transluminal Endoscopic Surgery. October 2005. *Surg Endosc* 2006; **20**: 329–333.

25. Association of Laparoscopic Surgeons of Great Britain and Ireland. *Statement on NOTES*. London: ALSGBI, 2008 <www.alsgbi.org>.

Shahab Siddiqi John Morlese Atique Imam

12

Radiological assessment of intestinal blood flow and function

The radiological assessment of gastrointestinal physiological function and blood flow is an expanding field. The conventional radiological reporting of features such as size and shape alone is becoming increasingly inadequate for diagnostic purposes. This has led to the development of imaging techniques which allow both physiological and functional interrogation and these techniques have the potential to improve diagnostic accuracy. This review is divided into two sections, the first concerning blood flow and the second functional section explores the radiological assessment of gastrointestinal motility and secretion. Improvements in older techniques are described as are potential future modalities.

BLOOD FLOW

Classically, radiology has been asked to assist the clinician in the diagnosis of overt intestinal haemorrhage and intestinal ischaemia. These investigative modalities look at blood vessels and visceral ischaemic changes. Newer techniques exploit the different ways blood and blood vessels act at the microscopic level to aid diagnostic discrimination in equivocal cross sectional imaging.

Shahab Siddiqi BSc FRCS (for correspondence)
Colorectal Fellow, Department of Colorectal Surgery, Castle Hill Hospital, Cottingham, East Yorkshire HU16 5JQ, UK. E-mail: shahab@doctors.org.uk

John Morlese BSc FRCR
Consultant Radiologist, Department of Radiology, Leicester Royal Infirmary, Infirmary Square, Leicester LE1 5WW, UK. E-mail: john.morlese@uhl-tr.nhs.uk

Atique Imam FRCS FRCR
Specialist Registrar in Radiology, Department of Radiology, John Radcliffe Hospital, Headley Way, Headington, Oxford OX3 9DU, UK. E-mail: atiqueimam777@hotmail.com

ACUTE GASTROINTESTINAL BLEEDING

Acute gastrointestinal (GI) bleeding remains a common clinical emergency. Upper and lower GI bleeding can be divided into those proximal or distal to the ligament of Treitz, respectively.[1] Timely and anatomically accurate localization of the bleeding source is vital in reducing mortality. Endoscopy is excellent at identifying upper GI causes and stratifying those patients who may benefit from surgical intervention. Colonoscopy is less useful due to poor views and decreased sensitivity for identifying the bleeding source.[2] Furthermore, neither technique will identify a small bowel source. Hence, radiological approaches have a central role in the diagnosis of major haemorrhage not detected by endoscopy.[3]

The available diagnostic modalities are discussed; however, the use of the techniques within a management algorithm varies with their availability and regional expertise. A management approach must be flexible to take this into account.

CATHETER ANGIOGRAPHY

Catheter angiography now has an extended therapeutic role, particularly in those patients who may not be fit for, or have had re-bled after, surgical intervention. In some specialist centres, it has become the primary therapeutic modality after endoscopy. Catheter angiography has a reported sensitivity ranging of 40–90% for the diagnosis of acute GI bleeding and is highly specific at 100%.[1,4] Haemorrhaging sites can be diagnosed and simultaneously treated with embolisation. Embolisation involves the intra-arterial release of substances in the feeding vessel as close to the bleeding point as possible. Stainless steel or platinum coils with polyester tufts, acrylic spheres, gelatin sponge and alcohol particles have been used alone or in combination as embolisation agents. Although, this technique is the gold standard for investigating acute GI bleeding, it has several associated disadvantages. Significant on-going haemorrhage of greater than 1 ml/min is required at the time of contrast injection. As new catheters have been introduced and expertise gained, highly selective mesenteric angiography is now possible. This has enabled accurate localisation of the haemorrhaging site at the lower required bleeding rate of 0.5 ml/min.[5] Even so, catheter angiography will not always find the bleeding source. It is also an invasive procedure that requires a highly skilled team which may not be readily available, particularly out of hours. Catheter angiography gives little clue about the pathological cause of the haemorrhage with the main exception of angiodysplasia. Furthermore, if an anomalous vascular supply is present and not examined, false-negative examinations can occur. An anomalous vasculature is common with a reported prevalence of up to 60%.[6] Therapeutic embolisation can also result in ischaemia and necrosis to the segment of treated bowel. The reported occurrence varies between 10–60% and there is a lesser rate of re-bleeding.[7,8] Neither should be considered a failure. The demarcated bowel can be targeted specifically by surgery rather than the usual gross resection in blind surgery. Even if embolisation does not stem the haemorrhage, a catheter left *in situ* will guide and limit resection. Specialist centres are increasingly using catheter angiographic therapy before surgery and some even in the situation of re-bleed after surgical under-running of a bleeding duodenal ulcer. No strong evidence is yet available to support this and there remains the increased risk of intestinal anastomotic dehiscence.

Key point 1

- Catheter angiography is diagnostic and can be therapeutic for major gastrointestinal haemorrhage.

COMPUTED TOMOGRAPHIC ANGIOGRAPHY

An ideal imaging technique should be simple, quick, non-invasive and widely available. Computed tomographic (CT) angiography is becoming such a procedure, albeit utilising intravenous iodine-based contrast agents to localise active bleeding points. Faster scans with thinner slices allow excellent multiplanar reformats of the CT data set, which can more clearly demonstrate the site of haemorrhage. Bleeding rates as low as 0.3 ml/min can be detected consistently.[9] CT angiography has a reported sensitivity and specificity of 91% and 99%, respectively.[10]

The CT angiography technique involves scanning approximately 25 s after a bolus of iodinated contrast has been given intravenously.[3,9] This corresponds with the late capillary phase of bowel wall enhancement and allows sufficient time for the contrast to pool in the bowel lumen if active bleeding is occurring. The major and mesenteric arterial vessels are also well visualised aiding localisation of the source vessel.[3,9] The whole abdomen and pelvis can be scanned in a matter of a few seconds and some units compare these images with an initial pre-contrast scan to determine subtle haemorrhage within the bowel lumen and exclude hyperdense artefacts more accurately.

CT angiography has the added benefit of potentially simultaneously diagnosing the cause of the bleeding. This may allow both interventional, radiological, lesion-directed treatment as well as pre-surgical planning. The disadvantages of CT angiography include nephrotoxicity and allergy due to the use of iodine-based contrast agents and the risks of radiation exposure. Despite the accuracy of CT angiography, the CT suite is an inappropriate place for an unstable patient; furthermore, a low cardiac output, resulting in poor opacification of the vessels, will decrease the sensitivity of the investigation.

Key points 2 and 3

- CT angiography is a strong diagnostic tool for acute gastrointestinal bleed and gives additional anatomical information about cause of bleed.

- Patients who are too haemodynamically unstable to undergo endoscopy are also too unstable to undergo CT.

RADIONUCLIDE IMAGING

Radionuclide imaging of GI bleeding has changed recently. Previously, single plane nuclear imaging was the norm, but the advent of multiple planar imaging allows a more accurate localisation of the bleeding source. The latter is known as single photon emission computed tomography (SPECT) and uses technetium-labelled red blood cells. It is up to 93% sensitive and 95% specific. It has the advantage over other techniques in that it can visualise lower rates of bleeding down to 0.05 ml/min anywhere in the GI tract.[11] Technetium-labelled red blood cell imaging can be performed over prolonged periods of time as opposed to the CT- and catheter-based angiographic methods. Disadvantages remain in that it can only be performed in specialist centres and anatomical localisation remains suboptimal.

CHOICE OF INVESTIGATION

The initial investigation largely depends on local expertise and availability. However, an unstable patient should not be taken to the endoscopy unit, CT suite or the nuclear medicine department. Catheter angiography is, therefore, more appropriate for the unstable case.

ACUTE MESENTERIC ISCHAEMIA

The mortality from acute mesenteric ischaemia remains high as the diagnosis is usually delayed and made at laparotomy. The major causes of acute mesenteric ischaemia include; superior mesenteric artery (SMA) embolus or thrombosis, mesenteric venous thrombosis and non-occlusive mesenteric vasoconstriction.[12] A high index of suspicion is required.

COMPUTED TOMOGRAPHY

CT is readily available for the investigation of the patient with an acute abdomen. Conventional radiological diagnosis is made using arterial phase CT scanning with the identification of the following features: extreme mucosal enhancement, thickened bowel wall, mesenteric oedema, intramural gas, portal venous gas, lack of SMA or superior mesenteric vein (SMV) enhancement and ischaemia of other organs.[2,13] The presence of at least one of these signs results in a 64% sensitivity and a 92% specificity for the detection of acute mesenteric ischaemia. It must be stressed, a normal CT scan does not exclude acute mesenteric ischaemia.

CATHETER ANGIOGRAPHY

Catheter angiography is the gold standard for the diagnosis of acute mesenteric ischaemia and allows pre-surgical planning. It has the advantage over CT in that it can be additionally therapeutic. There has been anecdotal evidence for the delivery of intra-arterial thrombolysis in treating mesenteric thrombus. Suction embolectomy, angioplasty and stenting are all recognised.[14,15] Catheter angiography has a reported 88% sensitivity for the diagnosis.[13] Angiographically, an embolus appears as a sharp cut-off of flow and thrombus appears as a more tapered occlusion.[16] Despite it being the gold standard in arterial ischaemia, in mesenteric vein thrombosis it is unreliable.[16,17] An unanswered question remains: what are the indications for catheter angiography? The authors believe only if CT signs are subtle, the diagnosis unsure, the patient is not compromised and catheter angiography immediately available should it be considered. Furthermore, revascularisation of gangrenous bowel can lead to major mucosal haemorrhage.

MAGNETIC RESONANCE IMAGING (MRI)

The use of MRI of the abdomen and magnetic resonance angiography (MRA) of mesenteric arteries has been reported in acute mesenteric ischaemia.[18] It is thought to be particularly effective for the diagnosis of mesenteric vein thrombosis.[16] Its role has yet to be defined and is rarely available out-of-hours, yet MRA has the potential to be as accurate as catheter angiography.

DUPLEX IMAGING OF GASTROINTESTINAL BLOOD FLOW

Duplex sonography is very good at diagnosing proximal SMA and coeliac axis stenosis or occlusion with a sensitivity of 92–100% for acute mesenteric ischaemia.[2] However, the inferior mesenteric artery (IMA) and distal SMA are difficult to visualise with ultrasonography due to the common limitations encountered with ultrasound such as the presence of overlying bowel gas. This problem can be negated by the use of intra-operative duplex scanning where the ultrasound probe can be placed directly on the vessels. This is especially useful if the operating surgeon is capable of embolectomy and vascular bypass.

CHOICE OF INVESTIGATION

Of the above, CT is the most commonly available and used modality. The best investigation to diagnose acute mesenteric ischaemia at an early stage is unclear because there is a significant false-negative rate with all approaches. Until this false negativity can be reduced, exploratory laparotomy will still have a major role.

Key point 4
- Computed tomography is the most readily available test for acute mesenteric ischaemia, but a normal scan does not exclude the diagnosis.

CHRONIC MESENTERIC ISCHAEMIA

Chronic mesenteric ischaemia is a difficult diagnosis to make as it presents with non-specific symptoms and signs. The symptoms include abdominal pain, poor appetite and weight loss. Even when the disease is suspected, confirming the diagnosis can be problematic. In the vast majority of cases, the cause of chronic mesenteric ischaemia is diffuse atherosclerotic disease.[19,20] Rarer causes include fibromuscular dysplasia, vasculitis and median arcuate syndrome.[21] General consensus is that two out of the three main mesenteric arteries must be involved.

CATHETER ANGIOGRAPHY

This is the criterion standard in which the presence of atherosclerotic disease in two mesenteric arteries either occlusion or stenosis, in the setting of symptoms, is considered diagnostic. However, imaging of the mesenteric arteries, particularly the more distal arteries, can be difficult.[19,20] Furthermore, the impact of collateral circulation is difficult to assess by angiographic means alone. Other modalities help including CT, MRA and duplex ultrasonography.[20,22] Unfortunately, these all have lower spatial resolution, are poorer at demonstrating more distal mesenteric artery stenosis, and also may fail to demonstrate which stenoses are functionally significant.[22]

NEW FUNCTIONAL MAGNETIC RESONANCE TECHNIQUES

In normal patients, the mesenteric blood flow increases after a meal; however, in patients with chronic mesenteric ischaemia, this postprandial augmentation of blood is delayed and diminished.[23] A new, non-invasive, functional MR method to assess mesenteric blood flow has been described. It involves demonstrating small bowel wall contrast enhancement.[24] This method utilises the fact that bowel wall enhancement after intravenous contrast administration is directly related to mesenteric blood flow. It also employs a stress component to the study in which the baseline blood flow values before a meal are compared with values after eating a standardised meal. This gives an estimate of the postprandial mesenteric reserve. This is the increase in mesenteric blood flow occurring after a meal. A reduction in this value is thought to be a more accurate measure of chronic mesenteric ischaemia. Different vascular territories can be interrogated in the same examination. At the same time, MRA of the coeliac trunk, SMA or IMA can be performed and correlated with the apparent bowel perfusion reserve measurements to determine which stenoses are functionally important.[24]

Key points 5 and 6

- Chronic mesenteric ischaemia remains a difficult clinical and radiological diagnosis to make.
- Catheter angiography remains gold standard for making the diagnosis and new functional tests may assist in diagnosis.

STRANGULATED HERNIAS

The differentiation between the need for immediate and urgent surgical intervention for an irreducible hernia is obvious if frankly gangrenous bowel is contained within the hernia sack. Radiology can help in those cases where it is not so clear. Contrast-enhanced CT and duplex ultrasound can both be used to determine the viability of bowel within a hernia. The single most significant independent predictor of a strangulated hernia was the reduced wall enhancement on CT which has a reported sensitivity of 56% and specificity of 94%.[25] Duplex ultrasound demonstrates peristalsis, oedematous bowel wall and the arterial blood supply.[26] Both investigations are not perfect and clinical suspicions should be followed.

CT DIFFERENTIATION OF BENIGN AND MALIGNANT COLORECTAL LESIONS

A common and important clinical problem is radiologically differentiating between acute diverticulitis and colon carcinoma.[27] Contrast-enhanced CT is the standard investigation in patients with suspected acute diverticulitis, the following radiological features suggesting the diagnosis: presence of diverticula, adjacent bowel wall thickening, stricturing, pericolic mesenteric fat stranding, paracolic lymph node enlargement, and abscess formation.[27] However, colorectal carcinoma may have similar imaging appearances and may co-exist with diverticular disease. In particular, bowel wall thickening, structuring and pericolic mesenteric fat stranding are present in both disease processes.

This has created a need for more physiological parameters to differentiate between these two entities. A large body of radiological research has targeted surrogate markers of angiogenesis. This is a cardinal feature of malignancy and has been routinely measured in brain tumours utilising CT and MR perfusion imaging.

These techniques have recently been applied to colorectal carcinoma where there is marked angiogenesis, allowing differentiation from both diverticular disease and acute diverticulitis in which angiogenesis is lacking. MR and CT perfusion can be used to estimate this difference.[27,28] The angiogenesis-derived new capillaries are abnormal with increased vessel wall leakiness, increased tortuosity and increased vessel numbers. These features can be estimated by the CT- or MR-derived parameters permeability, mean transit time and blood volume, respectively. Colorectal carcinoma is characterised by marked angiogenesis whilst diverticulitis is not. Significant differences were noted in patients with diverticular disease, diverticulitis and colorectal cancer.[28] Colorectal cancer was found to have increased blood volume and mean transit time and in comparison with non-inflamed diverticular disease. When compared with standard morphological features, perfusion was the most specific parameter for diagnosis of colorectal carcinoma.[28]

The utility of physiological assessments of disease is a large area of research in radiology. It is known that morphological changes such as size and shape alone cannot differentiate reliably between colorectal carcinoma and diverticular disease. In addition, new chemotherapeutic agents (such as the anti-angiogenic drugs) initially reduce the vascularity of a tumour without altering its size. Therefore, conventional morphological measurements will be insufficient to assess treatment response. CT and MR perfusion scans for colorectal disease could enter clinical practice in the near future if early reports are reproducible.

FUNCTIONAL RADIOLOGY

Radiology is becoming increasingly useful in the assessment of physiological function of the intestinal tract. Currently, breath tests, manometry and endoscopy are the mainstay, but radiology is especially useful in motility studies. It is evident that information from multiple investigative modalities is required to analyse function. However, it is hoped that radiology will allow the routine non-invasive analysis of GI function, previously the remit of a few specialist centres. Plain radiographs, videofluoroscopy and MRI are the main modalities utilised.

OESOPHAGEAL FUNCTION TESTING

Videofluoroscopy allows detailed examination of the movement of the oesophagus by repeated tests with radio-opaque food boluses. This complements other tests such as oesophageal manometry.[29] Computerised scintigraphic analysis of the movement of swallowed radiolabelled boluses can give quantitative information about the patterns of movement of material down the oesophagus, but barium radiology is better if performed well.[29] Normal transit takes 15 s with three distinct peaks. Diffuse oesophageal spasm is the main functional disorder which can be seen by imaging techniques. Classically, barium swallow shows beads of contrast in the distal oesophagus known as the corkscrew oesophagus, or sustained obliteration by contraction of the distal oesophagus.[30] However, this is only an intermittent finding and manometry is the main investigation.

GASTRIC FUNCTION AND EMPTYING

The measurement of gastric function and emptying is inexact and is influenced by gastric compliance, contractility and distal resistance. A single test will not provide sufficient information. Gastroparesis can occur in diabetic individuals, following gastric surgery and is associated with other conditions. A number of imaging tests can be utilised to analyse gastric function. The simplest involves the addition of small amounts of technetium and/or indium to simple foods which are then ingested. Real-time gamma scanning over the stomach allows gastric emptying to be measured. About 50% of gastric activity should empty in 1 h in a normal stomach, but errors can occur in measurement as the stomach and scanner can move.[31] Gastric barium emptying is less reliable unless the contrast is incorporated into food. Recently, MRI has been shown to be as good in analysing gastric emptying. Additional advantages of MRI are that gastric contractility and secretion can be investigated. However, this is still a research tool.[31,32]

INTESTINAL TRANSIT

Intestinal slow transit can be colonic or pan-intestinal. The differentiation is important as management paths diverge. A plain abdominal radiograph can confirm the presence of faecal material throughout the colon and allows measurement of the diameter of the small intestine and colon. This will exclude pseudo-obstruction and megacolon. Radionuclide techniques can be used to determine small-bowel transit by timing the appearance of counts over the caecum after oral ingestion. Estimates of colonic transit time can be measured with further readings. Normally, the orocaecal transit time is less than 90 min, but it is defined as abnormal only if it is > 6 h.[33,34] Improvements to this have been made by the use of enteric capsule s which only release the radioactive carbon once in the small bowel.[34]

Plain radiographs can help determine colonic transit times. Various methodologies are available involving the ingestion of small pieces of radio-opaque plastic and taking a plain abdominal radiograph after 5 days. The patient should not be taking any laxatives and the radiograph reveals the number of remaining markers and their distribution in the colon. Other methods include taking three differently shaped plastic objects on different days, but this provides little additional information. It may help distinguish those with a pelvic outflow obstruction, but others disagree.[35] In essence, transit is normal if < 80% markers are seen after 5 days.[33] MRI has been shown to be capable of analysing small and large bowel motility and function after ingestion of ispaghula labelled with a positive paramagnetic contrast agent. It can also measure small bowel contractility, bolus movement, secretion and absorption. The amount of time required in the scanner currently makes its use impractical.[31] However, its ability to analyse function as well as transit may make this a major future diagnostic tool.

VISCERAL SENSATION

Functional MRI has been used extensively recently to investigate brain function. The same technique has been translated to the bowel. It has the possibility to correlate visceral pain with physiological function in people with functional intestinal disorders. It has already shown different cerebral responses to GI stimulation in areas concerned with emotion and discrimination. Future developments of magnetic resonance spectography may even allow the monitoring of neurotransmitters in the enteric nervous system.[31]

DEFAECATING PROCTOGRAPHY AND ANAL SPHINCTERS

Defaecating proctography can be used to assess anorectal function if there are symptoms to suggest constipation, obstructive defaecation, rectal prolapse or anismus.[36] Others recently have suggested recto-anal intussusception is a common finding in individuals with faecal incontinence. It was found in 60% and they recommended proctography as a routine imaging modality in faecal incontinence.[37] Defaecation involves the co-ordination of the rectum, anus and pelvic floor. However, a fluoroscopic proctogram will only give luminal information and normal evacuation should take 5–40 s. The anorectal angle is 90° at rest and becomes more obtuse during defaecation. Rectoceles, enteroceles and intrarectal intussusception can also be identified.[36] A recent study has shown that a trans-labial ultrasound was well tolerated and could reveal rectoceles and intussusception. It was put forward as a screening test.[38]

Open MRI now allows dynamic MRI proctography by accommodating a sitting patient. The rectum is filled with semisolid labelled contrast marker, the patient is positioned sitting on a commode and sequences taken during defaecation. MRI proctography is now the gold standard as it allows analysis of the rectal wall for intussusception and rectocele, the anorectal angle, anal canal opening, pelvic floor movement and surrounding visceral structures.[36,39] Additionally, it provides excellent imaging of the anal sphincter with or without an endo-anal coil.[40] However, MRI proctography is not available in all centres.

Anal ultrasound is excellent in assessing the integrity of the sphincter complex. However, it cannot comment on the functional significance of any findings as an individual with complete sphincter disruption may be continent. Recently, three-dimensional dynamic anal ultrasound has been introduced. It may improve assessment and change an operative approach.[41] Three-dimensional ultrasound has also been used with the probe proximal to the anus to detect the same anorectal dysfunctions as seen by a defaecating proctogram.[42]

Key points 7 and 8

- Dynamic magnetic resonance imaging has become an excellent modality to investigate defaecatory disorders.

- The anal sphincters are accurately imaged by magnetic resonance imaging.

BILE SALTS AND MALABSORPTION

Bile salt malabsorption can be found after ileal resection, in diseases of the terminal ileum and in idiopathic bile salt malabsorption due to transporter defects. Small bowel bacterial overgrowth deconjugates bile salts which also impairs absorption and retention. A SeHCAT test uses orally administered radiolabelled selenohomocholic acid. A gamma camera measures whole body retention after 7 days. Excessive loss of bile salts gives a low retention value of 5% or less.[43]

SUMMARY

The explosion in imaging technology is improving diagnosis and increasingly permits simultaneous therapy. Newer techniques analyse function as well as morphology helping differentiate aetiology. In fact, radiology is increasing our physiological and anatomical understanding of the GI tract and pelvic floor.[44] Their place in a physician's diagnostic and therapeutic algorithm is yet to be established.

Key points for clinical practice

- Catheter angiography is diagnostic and can be therapeutic for major gastrointestinal haemorrhage.

continued on next page

Key points for clinical practice *(continued)*

- CT angiography is a strong diagnostic tool for acute gastrointestinal bleed and gives additional anatomical information about cause of bleed.

- Patients who are too haemodynamically unstable to undergo endoscopy are also too unstable to undergo CT.

- Computed tomography is the most readily available test for acute mesenteric ischaemia, but a normal scan does not exclude the diagnosis.

- Chronic mesenteric ischaemia remains a difficult clinical and radiological diagnosis to make.

- Catheter angiography remains gold standard for making the diagnosis and new functional tests may assist in diagnosis.

- Dynamic magnetic resonance imaging has become an excellent modality to investigate defaecatory disorders.

- The anal sphincters are accurately imaged by magnetic resonance imaging.

References

1. Lee EW, Laberge JM. Differential diagnosis of gastrointestinal bleeding. *Tech Vasc Intervent Radiol* 2004; **7**: 112–122.
2. Lefkovitz Z, Cappell MS, Lookstein R, Mitty HA, Gerard PS. Radiologic diagnosis and treatment of gastrointestinal hemorrhage and ischemia. *Med Clin North Am* 2002; **86**: 1357–1399.
3. Laing CJ, Tobias T, Rosenblum DI, Banker WL, Tseng L, Tamarkin SW. Acute gastrointestinal bleeding: emerging role of multidetector CT angiography and review of current imaging techniques. *Radiographics* 2007; **27**: 1055–1070.
4. Rahn III NH, Tishler JM, Han SY, Russinovich NA. Diagnostic and interventional angiography in acute gastrointestinal hemorrhage. *Radiology* 1982; **143**: 361–366.
5. Baum ST. Arteriographic diagnosis and treatment of gastrointestinal bleeding. In: Baum ST, Pentecost MJ. (eds) *Abram's angiography interventional radiology*. Philadelphia, PA: Lippincott, Williams & Wilkins, 2006.
6. Winston CB, Lee NA, Jarnagin WR *et al*. CT angiography for delineation of celiac and superior mesenteric artery variants in patients undergoing hepatobiliary and pancreatic surgery. *AJR Am J Roentgenol* 2007; **189**: W13–W19.
7. Burgess AN, Evans PM. Lower gastrointestinal haemorrhage and superselective angiographic embolization. *Aust NZ J Surg* 2004; **74**: 635–638.
8. Sheth R, Someshwar V, Warawdekar G. Treatment of acute lower gastrointestinal hemorrhage by superselective transcatheter embolization. *Indian J Gastroenterol* 2006; **25**: 290–294.
9. Kuhle WG, Sheiman RG. Detection of active colonic hemorrhage with use of helical CT: findings in a swine model. *Radiology* 2003; **228**: 743–752.
10. Junquera F, Quiroga S, Saperas E *et al*. Accuracy of helical computed tomographic angiography for the diagnosis of colonic angiodysplasia. *Gastroenterology* 2000; **119**: 293–299.
11. Zuckier LS. Acute gastrointestinal bleeding. *Semin Nucl Med* 2003; **33**: 297–311.
12. Oldenburg WA, Lau LL, Rodenberg TJ, Edmonds HJ, Burger CD. Acute mesenteric ischemia: a clinical review. *Arch Intern Med* 2004; **164**: 1054–1062.

13. Taourel PG, Deneuville M, Pradel JA, Regent D, Bruel JM. Acute mesenteric ischemia: diagnosis with contrast-enhanced CT. *Radiology* 1996; **199**: 632–636.
14. Gartenschlaeger S, Bender S, Maeurer J, Schroeder RJ. Successful percutaneous transluminal angioplasty and stenting in acute mesenteric ischemia. *Cardiovasc Intervent Radiol* 2008; **31**: 398–400.
15. Berland T, Oldenburg WA. Acute mesenteric ischemia. *Curr Gastroenterol Rep*ort 2008; **10**: 341–346.
16. Shih MC, Hagspiel KD. CTA and MRA in mesenteric ischemia: part 1, Role in diagnosis and differential diagnosis. *AJR Am J Roentgenol* 2007; **188**: 452–461.
17. Kirkpatrick ID, Kroeker MA, Greenberg HM. Biphasic CT with mesenteric CT angiography in the evaluation of acute mesenteric ischemia: initial experience. *Radiology* 2003; **229**: 91–98.
18. Yasuhara H. Acute mesenteric ischemia: the challenge of gastroenterology. *Surg Today* 2005; **35**: 185–195.
19. Sreenarasimhaiah J. Diagnosis and management of intestinal ischaemic disorders. *BMJ* 2003; **326**: 1372–1376.
20. Zacho HD, Abrahamsen J. Chronic intestinal ischaemia: diagnosis. *Clin Physiol Funct Imaging* 2008; **28**: 71–75.
21. Hagspiel KD, Angle JF, Spinosa DJ, Matsumoto AH. Mesenteric ischemia: angiography and endovascular interventions. In: Longo W, Peterson GJ, Jacobs DL. (eds) *Intestinal ischemia disorders: pathophysiology and management.* St Louis, MO: Quality Medical Publishing, 1999; 105–154.
22. Cognet F, Ben Salem D, Dranssart M *et al.* Chronic mesenteric ischemia: imaging and percutaneous treatment. *Radiographics* 2002; **22**: 863–879.
23. Burkart DJ, Johnson CD, Reading CC, Ehman RL. MR measurements of mesenteric venous flow: prospective evaluation in healthy volunteers and patients with suspected chronic mesenteric ischemia. *Radiology* 1995; **194**: 801–806.
24. Lauenstein TC, Ajaj W, Narin B *et al.* MR imaging of apparent small-bowel perfusion for diagnosing mesenteric ischemia: feasibility study. *Radiology* 2005; **234**: 569–575.
25. Jancelewicz T, Vu LT, Shawo AE, Yeh B, Gasper WJ, Harris HW. Predicting strangulated small bowel obstruction: an old problem revisited. *J Gastrointest Surg* 2009; **13**: 93–99.
26. Yu PC, Ko SF, Lee TY, Ng SH, Huang CC, Wan YL. Small bowel obstruction due to incarcerated sciatic hernia: ultrasound diagnosis. *Br J Radiol* 2002; **75**: 381–383.
27. Goh V, Halligan S, Hugill JA, Bassett P, Bartram CI. Quantitative assessment of colorectal cancer perfusion using MDCT: inter- and intraobserver agreement. *AJR Am J Roentgenol* 2005; **185**: 225–231.
28. Goh V, Halligan S, Taylor SA, Burling D, Bassett P, Bartram CI. Differentiation between diverticulitis and colorectal cancer: quantitative CT perfusion measurements versus morphologic criteria – initial experience. *Radiology* 2007; **242**: 456–462.
29. Kawai T, Yamagishi T. Comparison of investigation modalities for evaluation of esophageal peristaltic function. *J Clin Biochem Nutr* 2008; **42**: 185–190.
30. Levine MS, Rubesin SE, Laufer I. Barium esophagography: a study for all seasons. *Clin Gastroenterol Hepatol* 2008; **6**: 11–25.
31. Schwizer W, Fox M, Steingotter A. Non-invasive investigation of gastrointestinal functions with magnetic resonance imaging: towards an 'ideal' investigation of gastrointestinal function. *Gut* 2003; **52 (Suppl 4)**: iv34–iv39.
32. Treier R, Steingoetter A, Goetze O *et al.* Fast and optimized T1 mapping technique for the noninvasive quantification of gastric secretion. *J Magn Reson Imaging* 2008; **28**: 96–102.
33. Lin HC, Prather C, Fisher RS *et al.* Measurement of gastrointestinal transit. *Dig Dis Sci* 2005; **50**: 989–1004.
34. Hung GU, Tsai CC, Lin WY. Development of a new method for small bowel transit study. *Ann Nucl Med* 2006; **20**: 387–392.
35. Cowlam S, Khan U, Mackie A, Varma JS, Yiannankou Y. Validity of segmental transit studies used in routine clinical practice, to characterize defaecatory disorder in patients with functional constipation. *Colorectal Dis* 2008; **10**: 818–822.
36. Ganeshan A, Anderson EM, Upponi S *et al.* Imaging of obstructed defecation. *Clin Radiol* 2008; **63**: 18–26.

37. Collinson R, Cunningham C, D'Costa H, Lindsey I. Rectal intussusception and unexplained faecal incontinence: findings of a proctographic study. *Colorectal Dis* 2009; **11**: 77–83.
38. Perniola G, Shek C, Chong CC, Chew S, Cartmill J, Dietz HP. Defecation proctography and translabial ultrasound in the investigation of defecatory disorders. *Ultrasound Obstet Gynecol* 2008; **31**: 567–571.
39. Mortele KJ, Fairhurst J. Dynamic MR defecography of the posterior compartment: indications, techniques and MRI features. *Eur J Radiol* 2007; **61**: 462–472.
40. Tan E, Anstee A, Koh DM, Gedroyc W, Tekkis PP. Diagnostic precision of endoanal MRI in the detection of anal sphincter pathology: a meta-analysis. *Int J Colorectal Dis* 2008; **23**: 641–651.
41. Gravante G, Giordano P. The role of three-dimensional endoluminal ultrasound imaging in the evaluation of anorectal diseases: a review. *Surg Endosc* 2008; **22**: 1570–1578.
42. Murad-Regadas SM, Regadas FS, Rodrigues LV, Silva FR, Soares FA, Escalante RD. A novel three-dimensional dynamic anorectal ultrasonography technique (echodefecography) to assess obstructed defecation, a comparison with defecography. *Surg Endosc* 2008; **22**: 974–979.
43. Wildt S, Norby RS, Lysgard MJ, Rumessen JJ. Bile acid malabsorption in patients with chronic diarrhoea: clinical value of SeHCAT test. *Scand J Gastroenterol* 2003; **38**: 826–830.
44. Dobben AC, Felt-Bersma RJ, ten Kate FJ, Stoker J. Cross-sectional imaging of the anal sphincter in fecal incontinence. *AJR Am J Roentgenol* 2008; **190**: 671–682.

Mark A. Fox Andrew R. Moore
Safa Al-Shamma Anthony I. Morris

13

Cancer surveillance in Crohn's disease and ulcerative colitis

Colorectal cancer is the third most common cancer in the UK affecting approximately 1-in-20[1] of the general population and is the second leading cause of cancer-related death.

Long-standing ulcerative colitis[2] and Crohn's disease[3–5] confer a similarly increased risk of developing colorectal cancer than the average population. Although inflammatory bowel disease-associated colorectal cancer only constitutes 2% of all colorectal malignancy, it is a frequent cause of death in this population[6,7] with an alarming 1-in-6 deaths attributable to colorectal malignancy.[8]

Five-year survival rates vary dramatically depending upon the stage of the disease. For localised disease, 92% 5-year survival rate is expected, for regional disease 62%, and for metastatic disease just 7%.[9] Treatment of colorectal cancer is costly and not without considerable morbidity and mortality. Consequently, colorectal cancer prevention and detection at an early stage is one of the most important goals of modern healthcare.

Mark A. Fox MBChB MRCP
Specialist Registrar in Gastroenterology, Department of Medicine, Royal Liverpool University Hospital, Royal Liverpool and Broadgreen University Hospitals NHS Trust, Prescot Street, Liverpool L7 8XP, UK

Andrew R. Moore MBChB MRCP (for correspondence)
Specialist Registrar in Gastroenterology, Department of Medicine, Royal Liverpool University Hospital, Royal Liverpool and Broadgreen University Hospitals NHS Trust, Prescot Street, Liverpool L7 8XP, UK. E-mail: doctorandymoore@hotmail.com

Safa Al-Shamma MBChB MRCP
Specialist Registrar in Gastroenterology, Department of Medicine, Royal Liverpool University Hospital, Royal Liverpool and Broadgreen University Hospitals NHS Trust, Prescot Street, Liverpool L7 8XP, UK

Anthony I. Morris MSc MD FRCP
Honorary Professor in Gastroenterology at Liverpool and John Moores Universities, Department of Medicine, Royal Liverpool University Hospital, Royal Liverpool and Broadgreen University Hospitals NHS Trust, Prescot Street, Liverpool L7 8XP, UK

Patients with inflammatory bowel disease are advised to undergo periodic colonoscopic surveillance to detect dysplasia or asymptomatic cancer at a curable stage.

We discuss the rationale for surveillance and current guidelines in inflammatory bowel disease. Most evidence in the literature relates to ulcerative colitis; however, the subsequent recommendations apply to both ulcerative colitis and Crohn's disease.

INFLAMMATORY BOWEL DISEASE-ASSOCIATED COLORECTAL MALIGNANCY

LEVEL OF RISK

The magnitude of risk of colorectal cancer in inflammatory bowel disease remains the subject of debate. While older reports demonstrated a rapid increase in risk after 10 years of disease,[6,10] recent studies suggest that the increased risk is less pronounced.[11,12]

Cumulative colorectal cancer risk in ulcerative colitis was examined by meta-analysis of all published studies in 2001[6] and later in the 2006 review of the largest surveillance programme to date (St Mark's group).[13] The findings are summarised in Table 1.

The reasons for such an improvement in the risk of ulcerative colitis/colorectal cancer are unclear but may include improved control of mucosal inflammation through more extensive use of 5-aminosalicylates and the implementation of surveillance programmes with timely colectomy once dysplasia is detected.[14]

Key point 1

- Inflammatory bowel disease is associated with increased risk of colorectal malignancy.

RISK FACTORS

Several independent risk factors, outlined in Table 2, influence the risk of malignant transformation. The duration of disease (from onset of symptoms) and extent of colonic mucosal inflammation are most prominent.

Table 1 Colorectal cancer risk relative to duration of disease

Reference	Colorectal cancer (%) and duration of colitis				Annual CRC risk after 10 years
	10 years	20 years	30 years	40 years	
Eaden et al. (2001)[6]	2	8	18	–	0.5–1.0% per-year
Rutter et al. (2006)[13]	–	2.5	7.6	10.7	–

CRC, colorectal cancer

Table 2 Risk factors for the development of colorectal malignancy in inflammatory bowel disease

Disease duration (from onset of symptoms)[6,15]
Young age (especially < 20 years) at onset[16,17]
Disease extent (of mucosal inflammation)[10,11,18,19]
Family history of sporadic colorectal carcinoma[20]
Persistence of mucosal inflammation[5,19]
Primary sclerosing cholangitis[21,22]
Presence of inflammatory pseudopolyps[19]
Presence of strictures[23]

A multitude of studies have correlated the extent of inflammation, including backwash ileitis,[18] with the risk of colorectal cancer[10,11,18,19] and neoplasia reported in areas of microscopic involvement alone. Only 'extensive' colitis (beyond the splenic flexure) appears to confer significant long-term increased risk. There is no increased risk with proctitis while left-sided disease represents intermediate risk.[16,17] The presence of pseudopolyps, which can be considered a surrogate marker of severity of inflammation, has been associated with double the risk of neoplasia.[19]

Cancer is rarely encountered when disease duration is less than 8–10 years but, thereafter, the risk rises at 0.5–1.0% per annum.[6,15] Thus, patients with onset of colitis early in life are thought to have an increased risk.[6,16,17]

Key point 2

- Disease duration and extent are major risk factors for the development of colorectal malignancy in inflammatory bowel disease.

INFLAMMATORY BOWEL DISEASE-ASSOCIATED CARCINOGENESIS

Inflammatory bowel disease-associated colorectal carcinogenesis is characterised by a 'chronic inflammation–dysplasia–carcinoma' sequence,[24] which differs from the well known 'adenoma–carcinoma' sequence in sporadic-colorectal cancer – a concept first described by Muto *et al.* in 1975.[25]

Although the exact mechanisms underlying this transition remain poorly understood, we do know that the molecular pathway for this process differs from that of sporadic-colorectal cancers.

APC and RAS mutations are less commonly found in inflammatory bowel disease colorectal cancer. Chromosomal instability, possibly as a consequence of telomere shortening,[26] is a frequent finding in inflammatory bowel disease colorectal cancer patients as opposed to inflammatory bowel disease patients without colorectal cancer.[27] In contrast to sporadic-colorectal cancer, chromosomal instability can be detected in non-dysplastic mucosa throughout the affected colon and, hence, could be used to identify high-risk patients.

Microsatellite instability results from mutations or promoter hyper-methylation of DNA mismatch repair genes leading to errors in DNA replication and accumulation of DNA damage. It is present in the vast majority of patients with Lynch syndrome and also present in up to 20% of sporadic-colorectal cancer.[28,29] Evidence exists correlating disease activity with higher levels of microsatellite instability. Patients with tumours possessing a high degree of microsatellite instability have a more favourable prognosis than those whose tumours are microsatellite stable.[28,30]

Hypermethylation of genes has been demonstrated in dysplastic as well as normal colonic tissue in inflammatory bowel disease colorectal cancer but not in inflammatory bowel disease patients without dysplasia.[31] It is most pronounced in genes that would normally methylate with age but occurs earlier in inflammatory bowel disease colorectal cancer. Thus, colitis can be seen as a condition leading to premature colonic ageing, explaining the earlier onset of colorectal cancer in inflammatory bowel disease.[32]

COMPARISON WITH SPORADIC COLORECTAL CANCER

When compared to sporadic disease, inflammatory bowel disease colorectal cancer develops in individuals at a younger age[24] with higher rates of proximal[33] and synchronous primary lesions.[24]

The prognosis of inflammatory bowel disease colorectal cancer has generally been considered worse than sporadic colorectal cancer; however, this may not be valid. In a report from the Mayo Clinic, the 5-year survival rates were 54% and 53% in the inflammatory bowel disease colorectal cancer and sporadic colorectal cancer, respectively.[34]

SURVEILLANCE PROGRAMMES

Surveillance colonoscopy programmes have been developed with the aim of reducing mortality due to colorectal cancer while avoiding unnecessary prophylactic colectomy.

Table 3 Summary of the British Society for Gastroenterology guidelines (2002)[35]

- Surveillance colonoscopy should be undertaken during remission
- All patients should undergo initial screening after 8–10 years with re-assessment of disease extent
- Regular surveillance should begin after 8–10 years and 15–20 years from onset of symptoms for extensive (beyond the splenic flexure) colitis and left-sided disease, respectively
- A reducing surveillance interval, in the order of 3-2-1-yearly colonoscopy, should be offered in the 2nd-3rd-4th decade of disease, respectively, in extensive (beyond the splenic flexure) disease
- Subjects with concomitant primary sclerosing cholangitis require annual endoscopic evaluation
- 2–4 random biopsies should be sampled every 10 cm from the entire colon with additional samples of 'suspicious' areas on white-light imaging
- Dysplasia of any grade, confirmed by two expert pathologists, justifies colectomy
- Maintenance 5-aminosalicylate therapy should be encouraged.

In the UK, the British Society for Gastroenterology guidelines from 2002,[35] outlined in Table 3, provide the foundation for current practice. The European Crohn's and Colitis Organisation (ECCO) published the most recent evidence-based guidance in 2008.[36] We review these recommendations, explain their rationale and draw attention to areas of debate.

TIMING AND NATURE OF COLONOSCOPY

Histological interpretation, in particular differentiating inflammatory change from dysplasia, can be problematic in the setting of active disease; therefore; surveillance is best performed during clinical remission.[37]

The aim of colonoscopy is to interrogate as much of the colonic mucosa as possible. With a greater proportion of proximal colorectal cancer in inflammatory bowel disease,[33] full colonoscopy is paramount. Rapid caecal intubation followed by meticulous inspection on withdrawal is optimal.

INITIAL SCREENING COLONOSCOPY

Timing of initial screening, which is also used to re-assess disease extent, is determined chiefly by disease duration. All patients should undergo initial screening after 8–10 years, the point at which dysplasia and cancer appear with any consistency. Onset of antecedent colitic symptoms rather than actual diagnosis is thought to provide a better estimation of years at risk and, therefore, advised as the starting point.

Since colorectal cancer is recognised before 8-years of disease,[33,38,39] this starting point has recently been challenged. A Dutch group have shown that 20% of those with inflammatory bowel disease-associated colorectal cancer in The Netherlands were diagnosed before the recommended British starting points raising the question of whether earlier surveillance would have been effective.[39]

LONG-TERM SURVEILLANCE SCHEDULE

The surveillance schedule recommended (see Table 3) is the product of three factors. First, the mean time between the development of low-grade dysplasia and cancer, the lead time, is 3 years.[40,41] Testing at intervals exceeding this is discouraged.[40] Second, as the risk of developing colorectal cancer or dysplasia increases with time, the testing interval decreases with increasing disease duration.[40] Third, since the extent of disease correlates with the incidence of neoplasia, a later starting point is rational for left-sided disease.[41]

In left-sided disease, although there is no evidence, the British Society for Gastroenterology[35] recommends 5-yearly colonoscopy with interim flexible sigmoidoscopy. Proctitis (at screening colonoscopy) does not require further surveillance.

Furthermore, although there are isolated case reports of neoplastic pouch transformation, there is no evidence to support routine surveillance of the ileal mucosa in ulcerative colitis patients following proctocolectomy with ileal pouch-anal anastomosis (IPAA).[44]

More recently, since colorectal cancer has been observed within 2 years of surveillance colonoscopy,[33,45] ECCO recommends bi-annual colonoscopy in the second decade of disease and annual assessment thereafter.[36]

Some authors suggest that additional risk-factors for inflammatory bowel disease-associated colorectal cancer, for instance family history of sporadic colorectal cancer, should be incorporated into future guidelines to assist stratification of risk and hence impact on the surveillance interval.[39,46] Similarly, some authorities suggest that risk-reducing factors, such as macroscopically normal mucosa at colonoscopy, could be included in order to downgrade the surveillance schedule.[47]

There is no evidence in the literature recommending an upper age limit at which surveillance should be terminated. For now, this requires an individualised case-based decision.

PRIMARY SCLEROSING CHOLANGITIS

Patients with primary sclerosing cholangitis, including those post orthotopic liver transplant, represent a sub-group at higher overall risk of colorectal cancer[21,22] with an estimated cumulative risk of 9%, 31% and 50% after 10, 20 and 25 years of colitis, respectively.[48] In addition, colorectal cancer has been reported to occur early (median, 2.9 years) in the disease course[49] and, typically, subjects exhibit clinically quiescent pan-colitis making estimation of the onset of colitis difficult. For these reasons, a more intensive schedule with annual surveillance colonoscopy is recommended.[35,36]

Key point 3

- Those with inflammatory bowel disease-associated primary sclerosing cholangitis represent a particularly high-risk group.

BIOPSY SAMPLING – RANDOM VERSUS TARGETED APPROACH

Dysplasia can be present focally as well as diffusely. Evidence suggests a minimum of 33 pan-colonic biopsies are needed to secure a 90–95% sensitivity for the detection of dysplasia.[50,51]

The British Society for Gastroenterology[35] recommends multiple serial random biopsies (four every 10 cm) from the entire colon using conventional white-light imaging. This represents a compromise between sensitivity and cost in terms of procedure time, pathology workload and related morbidity. 'Suspicious' areas such as raised lesions, traditionally referred to as 'dysplasia-associated lesions or masses' in the context of colitis, should also be sampled.[35]

In recent years, there has been a shift from this random protocol to a targeted approach through implementation of optical techniques that enhance the detection of dysplastic epithelium. Of these, chromendoscopy has become most wide-spread and is recommended by ECCO.[36] This involves coating the colonic epithelium with a dye (such as methylene blue or indigo-carmine) to highlight subtle architectural changes in the mucosa. This not only improves the diagnostic yield for dysplasia[52-55] but may also reduce the burden on

Table 4 The modified Kudo criteria for the classification of colorectal crypt architecture *in vivo* using high magnification chromoscopic colonoscopy (HMCC).[58]

Pit type	Characteristics	Pit size (mm)
I	Normal, round pits	0.07 (± 0.02)
II	Stellar or papillary	0.09 (± 0.02)
III-S	Tubular pits. Round in shape, smaller than in type I	0.03 (± 0.01)
III-L	Tubular, large pits	0.22 (± 0.09)
IV	Sulcus/gyrus pattern, resembling the pattern found on the surface of the cerebrum	0.93 (± 0.32)
V	Pits of varied type and size, arranged irregularly	n/a

pathology as fewer biopsies are required. Crucially, in expert hands, chromendoscopy does not take significantly longer than standard colonoscopy;[37] however, colonoscopists do require appropriate training while guidelines exist to aid optimal performance.[56]

The characteristics of neoplastic lesions as defined by their pit pattern on stereomicroscopy were described as early as 1975[57] and can now be identified *in vivo* by high-magnification chromoscopic colonoscopy (HMCC). The correlation between the histological and the endoscopic techniques has been validated in large series.[58,59] The modified Kudo criteria, shown in Table 4, enable classification of colorectal lesions on HMCC according to their pit-pattern.[58]

A multitude of additional emerging endoscopic tools may aid in the visualisation of subtle abnormalities and even distinguish neoplastic from non-neoplastic lesions (*e.g.* narrow band imaging [NBI], autofluorescence imaging [AFI], endomicroscopy, confocal laser microscopy, and optical coherence tomography) but it remains to be seen to what extent these will be harnessed in practice.

Surveillance of those with multiple inflammatory pseudopolyps and impassable strictures, where adequate sampling is not feasible and chromendoscopy unhelpful, is clearly insensitive. Under these circumstances, the merits of prophylactic colectomy versus intensified surveillance should be discussed with patients.

Key point 4

- Optical techniques, like chromendoscopy, facilitate targeted biopsy sampling and improve the diagnostic yield for dysplasia but require additional operator training.

APPROACH TO DYSPLASIA

Dysplasia is pre-malignant and can arise in both flat and raised (DALM) mucosa. It is stratified as low-grade, high-grade or indefinite for dysplasia

Table 5 Colorectal cancer risk relative to nature of dysplastic lesion identified on surveillance colonoscopy

Type of dysplastic lesion		Magnitude of colorectal cancer risk
Morphology	Grade	
DALM	Any	• Colorectal cancer in 43% at immediate colectomy[60]
Flat	High-grade	• Colorectal cancer in 42–67% at immediate colectomy[33,60]
Flat	Low-grade	• Overall 9-fold future increased risk of colorectal cancer[61]
		• 54% progression to high-grade dysplasia or colorectal cancer at 5-years[33]

which impacts on the likelihood of concomitant malignancy and future transformation as depicted in Table 5.

Clearly, the finding of dysplasia carries substantial risk; once detected, the rationale for surveillance demands that proctocolectomy is performed. Consequently, and because inter-observer variation for the detection of dysplasia is high,[62] this finding should be confirmed by a second, independent, experienced, gastrointestinal pathologist.

Until recently, DALMs have been considered an absolute indication for colectomy. Some may, however, resemble sporadic adenomas and, in the absence of dysplasia in the adjacent flat mucosa, may be amenable to endoscopic resection with subsequent intensive 3–6 monthly surveillance.[36]

Key point 5

• All patients should be offered entry into a colonoscopic surveillance programme.

CHEMOPREVENTION

The persistence of mucosal inflammation promotes risk of colorectal cancer.[5,19] Several studies indicate that maintenance therapy with a 5-aminosalicylate, which is generally well tolerated, may reduce colorectal cancer risk[63–65] and is, hence, encouraged. In fact, the number-needed-to-treat to prevent one colorectal cancer may be as low as 7 patients with 30-years of disease.[66]

Since randomised studies[67] show a lower incidence of dysplasia and colorectal cancer in patients with ulcerative colitis-associated primary sclerosing cholangitis, chemoprevention with ursodeoxycholic acid is recommended by ECCO[36] to all patients with ulcerative colitis and primary sclerosing cholangitis.

EFFECTIVENESS OF SURVEILLANCE PROGRAMMES

Although patients with colitis are at increased risk of developing colorectal cancer, to date unequivocal evidence demonstrating a survival benefit of cancer surveillance programmes is lacking.[10] Patients should be aware that surveillance can not guarantee a reduced cancer risk but rather offers a reasonable chance of detecting early symptomless disease. Indeed, in the largest and most meticulous screening programme reported to date, 16 of 30 (53.3%) cancers were interval cancers.[13]

Nevertheless, cancers detected in surveillance programmes tend to be at an earlier stage than those detected outside surveillance and are associated with a better prognosis.

Key points 6–8

- Surveillance aims to detect dysplasia or asymptomatic cancer at a curable stage.
- Chemoprotective agents are well-tolerated and may reduce cancer risk.
- Surveillance is not fool-proof and can not guarantee early detection of colorectal carcinoma.

SMALL BOWEL MALIGNANCY IN CROHN'S DISEASE

Small bowel adenocarcinoma is a rare complication of small bowel Crohn's disease. Meta-analyses have suggested that the risk of developing small bowel adenocarcinoma is increased approximately 30-fold in patients with Crohn's disease.[68,69] As cancer in the small bowel can mimic the symptoms of acute inflammation or of stricturing disease, diagnosis prior to surgery has historically been difficult. As a result, the disease is often advanced at diagnosis and the outcome poor.[70]

Given the rarity of small bowel cancer and the challenges posed in examining this segment of intestine, surveillance is not routinely indicated. Current advice would be to consider early examination of the small intestine when symptoms prompt this.

A recent case control study found that the two groups in which small bowel adenocarcinoma was reduced were those patients who had small bowel resection and in those with long-term (> 2 years) use of aminosalicylates.[71] Despite these data, few clinicians would propose either small bowel resection or long-term 5-aminosalicylate use solely to ameliorate the risk of small bowel adenocarcinoma, though the study does promote the suggestion that on-going inflammation is the primary risk factor for developing malignancy.

Key points for clinical practice

- Inflammatory bowel disease is associated with increased risk of colorectal malignancy.
- Disease duration and extent are major risk factors for the development of colorectal malignancy in inflammatory bowel disease.

Continued on next page

Key points for clinical practice *(Continued)*

- Those with inflammatory bowel disease-associated primary sclerosing cholangitis represent a particularly high-risk group.

- Optical techniques, like chromendoscopy, facilitate targeted biopsy sampling and improve the diagnostic yield for dysplasia but require additional operator training.

- All patients should be offered entry into a colonoscopic surveillance programme.

- Surveillance aims to detect dysplasia or asymptomatic cancer at a curable stage.

- Chemoprotective agents are well-tolerated and may reduce cancer risk.

- Surveillance is not fool-proof and can not guarantee early detection of colorectal carcinoma.

References

1. Quinn MWH, Cooper N, Rowan S *et al*. Cancer atlas of the United Kingdom and Ireland 1991–2000. National Statistics, 2005.
2. Edwards FC, Truelove SC. The course and prognosis of ulcerative colitis. Part IV: carcinoma of the colon. *Gut* 1964; **5**: 15–22.
3. Ekbom A, Helmick C, Zack M *et al*. Increased risk of large-bowel cancer in Crohn's disease with colonic involvement. *Lancet* 1990; **336**: 357–359.
4. Sachar DB. Cancer in Crohn's disease – dispelling the myths. *Gut* 1994; **35**: 1507–1508.
5. Jess T, Gamborg M, Matzen P *et al*. Increased risk of intestinal cancer in Crohn's disease: a meta-analysis. *Gut* 2001; **48**: 526–535.
6. Eaden JA, Abrams K, Mayberry JF. The risk of colorectal cancer in ulcerative colitis: a meta-analysis. *Gut* 2001; **48**: 526–535.
7. Winawer SJ. Natural history of colorectal cancer. *Am J Med* 1999; **106**: 3S–6S, discussion 50S–51S.
8. Hurlstone DP, Brown S. Techniques for targeting screening in ulcerative colitis. *Postgrad Med J* 2007; **83**: 451–460.
9. Parker SL, Tong T, Bolden S *et al*. Cancer statistics, 1996. *CA Cancer J Clin* 1996; **65**: 5–27.
10. Collins PD, Mpofu C, Watson AJ, Rhodes JM. Strategies for detecting colon cancer and/or dysplasia in patients with inflammatory bowel disease. *Cochrane Database Syst Rev* 2006; **2**: CD000279.
11. Lakatos L, Mester G, Erdelyi Z *et al*. Risk-factors for ulcerative colitis-associated colorectal cancer in a Hungarian cohort of patients with ulcerative colitis: results of a population-based study. *Inflamm Bowel Dis* 2006; **12**: 205–211.
12. Winther KV, Jess T, Langholz E *et al*. Long-term risk of cancer in ulcerative colitis: a population-based cohort from Copenhagen County. *Clin Gastroenterol Hepatol* 2004; **2**: 1088–1095.
13. Rutter MD, Saunders BP, Wilkonson KH *et al*. Thirty-year analysis of a colonoscopic surveillance programme for neoplasia in ulcerative colitis. *Gastroenterology* 2006; **130**: 1030–1038.
14. Loftus EV. Epidemiology and risk factors for colorectal dysplasia and cancer in ulcerative colitis. *Gastroenterol Clin North Am* 2006; **35**: 517–531.
15. Ransohoff DF. Colon cancer in ulcerative colitis. *Gastroenterology* 1988; **94**: 1089–1091.

16. Gyde SN, Prior P, Allan RN *et al.* Colorectal cancer in ulcerative colitis: a cohort study of primary referral from three centres. *Gut* 1988; **29**: 206–217.

17. Ekbom A, Helmick C, Zack M *et al.* Ulcerative colitis and colorectal cancer. A population-based study. *N Engl J Med* 1990; **323**: 1228–1233.

18. Heuschen UA, Hinz U, Allemeyer *et al.* Backwash ileitis is strongly associated with colorectal carcinoma in ulcerative colitis. *Gastroenterology* 2001; **120**: 841–847.

19. Rutter MD, Saunders BP, Wilkinson KH *et al.* Severity of inflammation is a risk factor for colorectal neoplasia in ulcerative colitis. *Gastroenterology* 2004; **126**; 451–459.

20. Nuako KW, Ahlquist DA, Mahoney DW *et al.* Familial predisposition for colorectal cancer in chronic ulcerative colitis: a case-control study. *Gastroenterology* 1998; **115**: 1079–1083.

21. Brentnall TA, Haggitt RC, Rabinovitch PS *et al.* Risk and natural history of colonic neolasia in patients with primary sclerosing cholangitis and ulcerative colitis. *Gastroenterology* 1996; **110**: 331–338.

22. Kornfeld D, Ekbom A, Ihre T. Is there an excess risk for colorectal carcinoma in patients with ulcerative colitis and concomitant primary sclerosing cholangitis? A population based study. *Gut* 1997; **41**: 522–525.

23. Lashner BA, Turner BC, Bostwick DG *et al.* Dysplasia and cancer complicating strictures in ulcerative colitis. *Dig Dis Sci* 1990; **35**: 349–352.

24. Choi PM. Predominance of rectosigmoid neoplasia in ulcerative colitis and its implication on cancer surveillance. *Gastroenterology* 1993; **104**: 666–667.

25. Muto T, Bussey HJR, Morson BC. The evolution of cancer of the colon and rectum. *Cancer* 1975; **36**: 2251–2270.

26. O'Sullivan JN, Bronner MP, Brentnall TA *et al.* Chromosomal instability in ulcerative colitis is related to telomere shortening. *Nat Genet* 2002; **32**: 280–284.

27. Rabinovitch PS, Dziadon S, Brentnall TA *et al.* Pancolonic chromosomal instability precedes dysplasia and cancer in ulcerative colitis. *Cancer Res* 1999; **59**: 5148–5153.

28. Gryfe R, Kim H, Hsieh ET *et al.* Tumour microsatellite instability and clinical outcome in young patients with colorectal cancer. *N Engl J Med* 2000; **342**: 69–77.

29. Hampel H, Frankel DW, Martin E *et al.* Screening for the Lynch syndrome. *N Engl J Med* 2005; **352**: 1851–1860.

30. Wantanabe T, Wu TT, Catalano PJ *et al.* Molecular predictors of survival after neoadjuvant chemotherapy for colon cancer. *N Engl J Med* 2001; **344**: 1196–1206.

31. Issa JP, Ahuja N, Toyota M *et al.* Accelerated age-related CpG island methylation in ulcerative colitis. *Cancer Res* 2001; **61**: 3573–3577.

32. Greenstein AJ. Cancer in inflammatory bowel disease. *Mt Sinai J Med* 2000; **67**: 227–240.

33. Connell WR, Lennard-Jones JE, Williams CB *et al.* Factors affecting the outcome of endoscopic surveillance for cancer in ulcerative colitis. *Gastroenterology* 1994; **107**: 933–944.

34. Delaunoit T, Limburg PJ, Goldberg RM *et al.* Colorectal cancer prognosis among patients with inflammatory bowel disease. *Clin Gastroenterol Hepatol* 2006; **4**: 335–342.

35. Eaden JA, Mayberry JF. Colorectal cancer screening: guidelines for screening and surveillance of asymptomatic colorectal cancer in patients with inflammatory bowel disease. *Gut* 2002; **51 (Suppl V)**: v10–v12.

36. Biancone L, Michetti P, Travis S *et al.* European evidence-based consensus on the management of ulcerative colitis: special situations. *J Crohn's Colitis* 2008; **2**: 63–92.

37. Riddell RH, Goldman H, Ransohoff DF *et al.* Dysplasia in inflammatory bowel disease: standardised classification with provisional clinical applications. *Hum Pathol* 1983; **14**: 931–966.

38. Bernstein CN. Low-grade dysplasia in ulcerative colitis. *Gastroenterology* 2004; **127**: 950–956.

39. Lutgens MWMD, Vleggaar FP, Schipper MEI *et al.* High frequency of early colorectal cancer in inflammatory bowel disease. *Gut* 2008; **57**: 1246–1251.

40. Lashner BA, Hanauer SB, Silverstein MD. Optimal timing of colonoscopy to screen for cancer in ulcerative colitis. *Ann Intern Med* 1988; **108**: 274–278.

41. Shapiro BD, Goldblum JR, Husain A *et al*. The role of p53 mutations in colorectal cancer surveillance for ulcerative colitis. *Gastroenterology* 1997; **112**: A1089.

42. Lashner BA, Watson AJM, McDonald J *et al*. *Evidence-based gastroenterology and hepatology*. London: BMJ Books, 2000; 221–229.

43. Riddell RH. Screening strategies in colorectal cancer. *Scan J Gastroenterol Suppl* 1990; **175**: 177–184.

44. Herline AJ, Meisinger LL, Rusin LC *et al*. Is routine pouch surveillance for dysplasia indicated for ileoanal pouches? *Dis Colon Rectum* 2003; **46**: 156–159.

45. Lim CH, Dixon MF, Vail A *et al*. Ten-year follow-up of ulcerative colitis patients with and without low-grade dysplasia. *Gut* 2003; **52**: 1127–1132.

46. Bernstein CN. Surveillance programmes for colorectal carcinoma in inflammatory bowel disease: have we got it right? *Gut* 2008; **57**: 1194–1196.

47. Rutter MD, Saunders BP, Wilkinson KH *et al*. Cancer surveillance in longstanding ulcerative colitis: endoscopic appearances help predict cancer risk. *Gut* 2004; **53**: 1813–1816.

48. Broome U, Lofberg R, Veress B *et al*. Primary sclerosing cholangitis and ulcerative colitis. Evidence for increased neoplastic potential. *Hepatology* 1995; **22**: 1404–1408.

49. Shetty K, Rybick L, Brzezinski A *et al*. The risk for cancer or dysplasia in ulcerative colitis patients with primary sclerosing cholangitis. *Am J Gastroenterol* 1999; **94**: 1643–1649.

50. Blackstone MO, Riddell RH, Rogers G *et al*. Dysplasia-associated lesion or mass (DALM) detected by colonoscopy in longstanding ulcerative colitis: an indication for colectomy. *Gastroenterology* 1981; **80**: 366–374.

51. Brostrom O, Lofberg R, Ost A *et al*. Cancer surveillance of patients with long-standing ulcerative colitis: a clinical, endoscopical and histological study. *Gut* 1986; **27**: 1408–1413.

52. Kiesslich R, Fritsch J, Holtmann M *et al*. Methylene blue aided chromendoscopy for the detection of intra-epithelial neoplasia and colon cancer in ulcerative colitis. *Gastroenterology* 2003; **124**: 880–888.

53. Rutter MD, Saunders BP, Schofiels G *et al*. Pancolonic indigo carmine dye spraying for the detection of dysplasia in ulcerative colitis. *Gut* 2004; **53**: 256–260.

54. Hurlstone DP, Sanders DS, McAlindon ME *et al*. High-magnification chromoscopic colonoscopy for the detection and characterisation of intraepithelial neoplasia in ulcerative colitis: a prospective evaluation. *Endoscopy* 2005; **37**: 1186–1192.

55. Matsumoto T, Nakamura S, Jo Y *et al*. Chromoscopy might improve diagnostic accuracy in cancer surveillance for ulcerative colitis. *Am J Gastroenterol* 2003; **98**: 1827–1833.

56. Kiesslich R, Neurath MF. Surveillance colonoscopy in ulcerative colitis: magnifying chromoendoscopy in the spotlight. *Gut* 2004; **53**: 165–167.

57. Kosaka T. Clinico-pathological study of the minute elevated lesion of the colorectal mucosa. *J Jpn Soc Coloproctol* 1975; **28**: 218–226.

58. Kudo S, Rubio CA, Teixeira CR *et al*. Pit pattern in colorectal neoplasia: endoscopic magnifying view. *Endoscopy* 2001; **33**: 367–373.

59. Hurlstone DP, Cross SS, Adam I *et al*. Efficacy of high magnification chromoscopic colonoscopy for the diagnosis of neoplasia in flat and depressed lesions of the colorectum: a prospective analysis. *Gut* 2004; **53**: 284–290.

60. Bernstein CN, Shanahan F, Weinstein WJ *et al*. Are we telling patients the truth about surveillance colonoscopy in ulcerative colitis? *Lancet* 1994; **343**: 71–74.

61. Thomas T, Abrams KA, Robinson RJ *et al*. Cancer risk of low-grade dysplasia in chronic ulcerative colitis: a systematic review and meta-analysis. *Aliment Pharmacol Ther* 2007; **25**: 657–668.

62. Odze RD, Goldblum J, Noffsinger A *et al*. Interobserver variability in the diagnosis of ulcerative colitis-associated dysplasia by telepathology. *Mod Pathol* 2002; **15**: 379–386.

63. Eaden JA, Abrams K, Ekbom A *et al*. Colorectal cancer prevention in ulcerative colitis: a case-control study. *Aliment Pharmacol Ther* 2000; **14**: 145–153.

64. Pinczowski D, Ekbom A, Baron J *et al*. Risk factors for colorectal cancer in patients with ulcerative colitis: a case-control study. *Gastroenterology* 1994; **107**: 117–120.

65. Moody GA, Jayanthi V, Probert CSJ *et al*. Long-term therapy with sulphasalazine

protects against colorectal cancer in ulcerative colitis: a retrospective study of colorectal cancer risk and compliance with treatment in Leicestershire. *Eur J Gastroenterol Hepatol* 1996; **8**: 1179–1183.

66. Munkholm P, Loftus EV, Reinacker-Schick N *et al*. Prevention of colorectal cancer in inflammatory bowel disease: value of screening and 5-aminosalicyates. *Digestion* 2006; **73**: 11–19.

67. Pardi DS, Loftus EV, Kremers WK *et al*. Ursodeoxycholic acid as a chemopreventative agent in patients with ulcerative colitis and primary sclerosing cholangitis. *Gastroenterology* 2003; **124**: 889–893.

68. von Roon AC, Reese G, Teare J, Constantinides N, Darzi AW, Tekkis PP. The risk of cancer in patients with Crohn's disease. *Dis Colon Rectum* 2007; **50**: 839–855.

69. Canavan C, Abrams KR, Mayberry J. Meta-analysis: colorectal and small bowel cancer risk in patients with Crohn's disease. *Aliment Pharmacol Ther* 2006; **23**: 1097–1104.

70. Dossett LA, White LM, Welch DC *et al*. Small bowel adenocarcinoma complicating Crohn's disease: case series and review of the literature. *Am Surg* 2007; **73**: 1181–1187.

71. Piton G, Cosnes J, Monnet E *et al*. Risk factors associated with small bowel adenocarcinoma in Crohn's disease: a case-control study. *Am J Gastroenterol* 2008; **103**: 1730–1736.

Jonathan K. Pye Sarah Cheslyn-Curtis

14

Delivery of general paediatric surgery in the 21st century

The future delivery of general paediatric surgery in local UK hospitals is heading for a crisis unless action is taken now.[1,2] Training in general paediatric surgery used to be part of the general education of the general surgeon and was provided in most district general hospitals (DGHs) throughout the UK. As subspecialisation developed within general surgery, this included general paediatric surgery with fewer surgeons in each DGH doing the elective surgery. In consequence, exposure to general paediatric surgery has been greatly reduced and training in the DGH is now minimal. Furthermore, the surgeons currently providing a general paediatric surgery service are approaching retirement with no-one to follow in their footsteps. This article outlines the current delivery of general paediatric surgery and discusses some of the potential ways forward.

> **Key points 1**
> - The delivery of general paediatric surgery is approaching a crisis. There is time to avert that crisis if action is taken now.

WHAT IS GENERAL PAEDIATRIC SURGERY?

General paediatric surgery is the surgery of the minor and intermediate conditions of childhood which require the support facilities that are present in

Jonathan K. Pye MBBS LRCP MRCS (for correspondence)
Consultant Surgeon, Department of Surgery, Wrexham Maelor Hospital, Croesnewydd Road,
Wrexham LL13, 7TD, UK. E-mail: jk.pye@zen.co.uk

Sarah Cheslyn-Curtis MBBS MS FRCS(Eng) FRCS(Gen)
Consultant Pancreatobiliary and General Paediatric Surgeon, Luton and Dunstable Hospital, Luton
LU6 2LH, UK and Royal Free Hospital, London NW3 2QG, UK

most DGHs. There is a clear distinction between general paediatric surgery and paediatric surgery. Paediatric surgery is the treatment of the conditions of childhood that require specialised surgery and support, and which are appropriately concentrated in 23 highly specialised centres. These focus on neonates, infants, children with congenital and acquired problems and the malignancies of childhood.

There is agreement[3] that elective general paediatric surgery is the management of, and surgery for, children with inguinal and umbilical hernias, undescended testis, conditions of the foreskin, minor ano-rectal conditions and excision of lesions of the skin and subcutaneous tissues. Emergency general paediatric surgery includes conditions that cause acute abdominal pain such as appendicitis, management of acute scrotal pain, incision and drainage of subcutaneous abscesses, managing children involved in trauma, and suturing skin lacerations. Some units manage infantile hypertrophic pyloric stenosis and intestinal obstruction caused by intussusception but, as these conditions occur in the younger age group, there is often limited experience in specialties such as anaesthetics and radiology to treat these conditions.

General paediatric surgery is mostly carried out by general surgeons in addition to their main adult surgical subspecialty; in some hospitals, urologists provide the service. There are increasing numbers of paediatric surgeons who provide general paediatric surgery on an out-reach or 'hub-and-spoke' basis in the DGH.[2] This provision varies from out-patient clinics being done in the DGH with children travelling to the paediatric centre for their surgery, to the surgeon travelling to the DGH to operate as well as for the out-patient work. In an average-sized DGH, the caseload is relatively modest and may amount to 1 or 2 sessions per week. This, therefore, adds little to the adult workload of the surgeon concerned and provides some variety to their clinical activities.

WHAT IS THE CRISIS?

Over the past decade, the emphasis on the delivery of surgical care has changed. There has been a major move towards subspecialisation and away from true general surgery. The emergency cases bind general surgery together, but elective work has become increasingly specialised and surgeons are working in a much narrower field of expertise. The training of surgeons has followed this change but the reduction in the hours of work has dramatically cut the time available in which to train registrars and for them to absorb the quantity of knowledge that formed the bedrock of most general surgeons who became consultants 10 or 15 years ago.

Over the past decade, exposure of trainees to general paediatric surgery has diminished substantially. Surgical trainees have focused on their main subspecialty for elective surgery. They are required to be on the emergency surgical rota[4] in order to manage the unselected emergency intake. The European Working Time Directive (EWTD) is due to come into full force in August 2009 which makes the learning week very short for surgical trainees to learn their craft. In 2004, additional training slots in paediatric surgery for general surgical trainees were funded to try to enhance training in general paediatric surgery; however, in almost every Deanery, trainees have been reluctant to take up the offer of training places in tertiary paediatric centres.

The main reason for this is that it eats into the short time available for learning their main clinical subspecialty. As a result, there is now a generation of trainees that are barely aware of general paediatric surgery as an additional subspecialty, have not trained in general paediatric surgery and, therefore, are not in a position to offer this as a surgical service when they reach the level of a trained surgeon.

Key points 2

- Elective general paediatric surgery is delivered locally in 66% of district general hospitals in the UK by general surgeons, urologists and paediatric surgeons.

All general surgical trainees are trained in the management of the 'acute' abdomen and to explore the scrotum for testicular pain. These skills are generic and apply to children as well as to adults. In this way, general paediatric surgery provision for the emergency cases in the older child can probably be maintained at the DGH. Anaesthetists are an important factor in the delivery of general paediatric surgery. During training, they all do a module of paediatric anaesthesia. Advice from the Royal College of Anaesthetists is that all 'adult' anaesthetists are expected to be able to anaesthetise children over the age of 5 years.[5] Those that undertake children's anaesthesia in the DGH are not expected to anaesthetise those less than 44 weeks' gestation, but even this would be exceptional in most DGHs with the lower age limit often being 2 years. As there is a general on-call rota for anaesthetists, it can not be expected that there will be particular expertise available each day of the week for paediatric emergencies. In over half (52.5%) of DGHs, emergencies are looked after by the general surgeons on call with a lower age limit of either 5 or 8 years depending on the hospital. A quarter of DGHs currently manage emergencies down to the age of 2 years.[2] The lower age limit is mainly dictated by anaesthetists as well as some surgeons, who may not be confident to manage children under the age of 5 years. Transfer out to a tertiary centre is very important when the expertise of the local clinicians is exceeded. Examples where early preparation for transfer should be a priority include major trauma, preterm infants and neonates except where local expertise is sufficient and available. Surgeons providing general paediatric surgery must be trained in advanced paediatric life support (APLS), and members of trauma teams must be fully trained in paediatric life support (PLS) with the necessary facilities available for full resuscitation and surgery if required. Children with multiple trauma should be transferred out as most will require paediatric intensive care unit facilities.

There has been a trend for general paediatric surgery to move away from the DGH into tertiary centres.[1,6] The tertiary centres, however, are not equipped to accommodate the volume of cases carried out across the UK. A recent survey in England, Wales and Northern Ireland identified that 138 DGHs (66%) provide elective general paediatric surgery, 147 (70%) provide emergency general paediatric surgery and in 63 DGHs (30%) there is no general paediatric surgery provision. There are approximately 23,000 elective

Table 1 The 2004–2005 statistics for children aged from 0–16 years (England)

Specialty	Total patients	Admissions	FCEs
Paediatric surgery	45,518	51,952	55,941
General surgery	48,865	51,041	53,824
ENT surgery	96,823	105,252	106,580
Trauma and orthopaedic surgery	74,128	86,773	89,989
Oral and maxillofacial surgery	4789	4885	5059
Oral surgery	45,296	47,035	47,309
Plastic surgery	32,154	36,009	36,530
Urology	14,270	16,326	16,985
Neurosurgery	4605	6659	7031
Cardiothoracic surgery	3655	2845	4808
Ophthalmology	16,866	19,867	20,003
Total	386,969	428,644	444,059

Source: UK Department of Health Hospital Episode Statistics.
FCEs, finished consultant episodes.

general paediatric surgery operations done outside the tertiary centres every year. Table 1 illustrates the workload by 'finished consultant episodes' taken from hospitals in England. These data include the 23 paediatric tertiary centres but, nevertheless, show that there is a considerable workload. Currently, there are 139 paediatric surgeons in the whole of the UK including Scotland. It can readily be seen that to incorporate the work from 138 DGHs into 23 tertiary centres is where the problem lies.

Looking to the future, 86% of the 138 hospitals currently doing general paediatric surgery said they could continue for another 5–10 years.[2] This leaves an opportunity to secure the future of general paediatric surgery in local hospitals if action is taken now.

LOOKING TO THE FUTURE

To address the future need requires three parallel actions. First, is to decide which model of general paediatric surgery provision is to be supported. Second, is to stimulate the training of surgeons and anaesthetists to look after these children. Third, is to encourage the purchasers and providers of healthcare that this is a priority and to allow sustainability for the next generations to be built in.

There is a powerful argument for keeping minor and intermediate level cases close to home so long as the surgeons and anaesthetists have been properly trained in general paediatric surgery and they have sufficient throughput to maintain competence. The local population wants it, the politicians want it and the paediatric tertiary centres not only cannot accommodate the additional workload, but they are unlikely to be able to increase their manpower and resources to do so. Even if the additional volume of cases could be accommodated in the tertiary centres, the paediatric surgeons do not want their specialist workload diluted by general paediatric surgery as it would increase the access time for all cases including the complex, specialist cases. It would also reduce the specialist training opportunities for their trainees.

Key points 3

- General paediatric surgery is a low-volume, 'special interest' caseload in each district general hospital that can be delivered in addition to a surgeon's main surgical subspecialty.

Purchasers of healthcare can enable the correct model by stipulating the standards of care they expect for the children on whose behalf they commission services. Also, the healthcare providers, which are mainly the hospital trusts, can inform the debate by advertising for consultant posts with an interest in general paediatric surgery in addition to the main surgical subspecialty they want for their hospital. This will give a signal to the trainees that there is benefit in obtaining training in general paediatric surgery as well as in their chosen subspecialty. Clinicians need evidence of a career pathway before they will invest the time in training for general paediatric surgery, and seeing that trusts are looking for general paediatric surgery surgeons will give that evidence.

MANPOWER

Manpower implications are important to take into consideration when deciding which model to adopt. A possible model is for paediatric surgeons to deliver general paediatric surgery on an out-reach basis. The problem with this model is that there are not enough paediatric surgeons to cover the hospitals that currently do general paediatric surgery. There would have to be a marked increase in the paediatric surgical manpower of over 100 in the next few years to cover the shortfall in general paediatric surgery provision. The current economic climate makes it highly unlikely that funding would be available to increase the paediatric surgical establishment to the level required. Even if that was possible, the volume of cases in any one DGH is not enough for a full-time appointment. Another model would be a joint appointment between the DGH and a tertiary paediatric centre. This model does exist in some parts of the UK. One difficulty that has been encountered is that the anaesthetists at the DGH do not all have the confidence to anaesthetise young children. The purpose of having expertise available locally is to carry out the necessary operations locally to avoid overburdening the tertiary centre. If the paediatric surgeon is unable to operate locally and has to take the children back to the tertiary centre, that defeats the object of the arrangement. Emergency cover also creates problems. The surgeon will not be able to provide 24-h cover 7 days a week. He or she is likely to be on the emergency rota for the tertiary centre rather than the DGH, leaving the DGH without their expertise locally.

Key points 4

- General paediatric surgery is an interesting and worthwhile addition to the subspecialty skills of a surgeon and will be required in many district general hospitals.

The majority of general paediatric surgery is carried out by general surgeons, with some urologists and some paediatric surgeons. The model that does not require any increase in manpower is to have general surgeons with urologists to continue to provide general paediatric surgery. The requirement for this to occur is an increase in the number of general surgeons and urologists being trained in general paediatric surgery. The two advantages of this model are that: (i) general paediatric surgery, both elective and emergency, could be kept in the local hospital; and (ii) there would be no manpower implications because the surgeons will be appointed for their main adult specialty and general paediatric surgery will be an additional skill that they would bring.

TRAINING AND EDUCATION

It is important that all trainees have some exposure to general paediatric surgery as most will have to manage children in the emergency setting. Few trainees currently obtain that exposure, so a fresh emphasis on the direction of training to incorporate general paediatric surgery is needed. The previous recommendation that general paediatric surgery training should only take place in a tertiary paediatric centre has been relaxed.[1] It is accepted that a minimum of 6 months of training in general paediatric surgery can be provided in a DGH with an experienced general paediatric surgery surgeon who has a sufficient caseload to give effective training. It can also be given in a paediatric centre or a combination of the two. An additional 6 months can be undertaken either in another DGH or in a paediatric centre for those that show inclination and aptitude for this surgery.[4] In order to identify those that may wish to take general paediatric surgery further, the surgeons who undertake general paediatric surgery need to be actively encouraged to teach, so that there is a greater awareness of general paediatric surgery among trainees. At the time of writing (December 2008), the Children's Surgical Forum of The Royal College of Surgeons of England is actively investigating which individuals and hospitals would be suitable to be approved for general paediatric surgery training as a step forward to resolve this issue. It may well be that there will be a network arrangement in each region for the programme director of higher surgical training to access. The detail is bound to differ between regions because the geography of each region and availability of paediatric tertiary centres varies across the UK. The length of time required to learn general paediatric surgery techniques is relatively short but achievable as the surgical skills required are directly transferable from adult surgery. Part of the training in general paediatric surgery is learning how to handle children and their families and other issues specific to children such paediatric life support and child protection.

Key points 5

- Training schemes are currently being devised to allow general paediatric surgery to continue to be delivered locally, for the benefit of children and their families.

PURCHASERS OF HEALTHCARE

The purchasers of healthcare also have a part to play. The main purchasing of healthcare in England is through the Strategic Health Authorities, in Wales through the Welsh Assembly Government and in Northern Ireland through the Department of Health, Social Services and Public Safety. These organisations must recognise the need for the local provision of minor and intermediate level care for their children. This is different from the organisational strategies that are essential for specialist care or for a system to cope with major trauma in children. Recognition of the difference between the two, and recognition of the impending crisis in the provision of general paediatric surgery is the key to proper strategic development. The healthcare providers, who are mainly the NHS hospital trusts, must play their part too. They should actively advertise for an additional interest in general paediatric surgery when seeking surgeons for their main subspecialty expertise. This will give the signal to trainees that learning how to manage general paediatric surgery is needed and will be welcomed when they have completed their surgical training.

SUMMARY

The UK is facing a crisis in the provision of general paediatric surgery. There are two main reasons underpinning this. First, is that many of the surgeons who currently provide general paediatric surgery are approaching retirement, and second, that surgical trainees are not being trained in general paediatric surgery. General paediatric surgery is a low-volume, interesting addition to the armamentarium of a surgeon. It gives variety in a surgical career and provides a service to the local population. If the ability to treat children locally disappears, we are likely to see children and their families having to travel to tertiary units for their treatment. General paediatric surgery is done in addition to the surgeon's main surgical subspecialty and, therefore, does not require an increase in the manpower establishment for an individual hospital. The key to avoiding the crisis is to increase the exposure of trainees to paediatric surgery and to train them in the DGH environment with or without input from a tertiary unit.

Key points for clinical practice

- The delivery of general paediatric surgery is approaching a crisis. There is time to avert that crisis if action is taken now.

- Elective general paediatric surgery is delivered locally in 66% of district general hospitals in the UK by general surgeons, urologists and paediatric surgeons.

- General paediatric surgery is a low-volume, 'special interest' caseload in each district general hospital that can be delivered in addition to a surgeon's main surgical subspecialty.

(continued)

Key points for clinical practice (continued)

- General paediatric surgery is an interesting and worthwhile addition to the subspecialty skills of a surgeon and will be required in many district general hospitals.

- Training schemes are currently being devised to allow general paediatric surgery to continue to be delivered locally, for the benefit of children and their families.

References

1. The Royal College of Surgeons of England. *Surgery for Children. Delivering a First Class Service.* Report of the Children's Surgical Forum. London: RCSE, 2007.
2. Pye JK. Survey of general paediatric surgery provision in England, Wales and Northern Ireland. *Ann R Coll Surg Engl* 2008; **90**: 193–197.
3. Crean P, Wilkins D, Boston V, Hamilton P, Smith JA. *Joint Statement on General Paediatric Surgery provision in District General Hospitals on behalf of the Association of Paediatric Anaesthetists, the Association of Surgeons for Great Britain and Ireland, the British Association of Paediatric Surgeons, the Royal College of Paediatrics and Child Health and the Senate of Surgery for Great Britain and Ireland.* 2006 <www.rcseng.ac.uk/service_delivery/children2019s-surgical-forum/documents/Aug%2006%20Joint%20statement%20GPS.pdf>.
4. *Intercollegiate Surgical Curriculum Project.* 2007 <www.iscp.ac.uk>.
5. The Royal College of Anaesthetists. *Guidelines for the Provision of Paediatric Anaesthetic Services.* 2004 <www.rcoa.ac.uk>.
6. Cochrane H, Tanner S. *Trends in Children's Surgery 1994–2005 Statistical Report.* 2007 <www.dh.gov.uk>.

Christopher Khoo

15

New techniques in plastic surgery

Plastic surgery has always been broadly based, supporting innovations in surgical techniques in areas which overlap with other surgical disciplines. This article sets out some recent developments in the key areas of breast surgery, facial reconstruction, wound healing and tissue repair, and current developments in the applications, design and monitoring of tissue flaps.

BREAST SURGERY: POST MASTECTOMY RECONSTRUCTION

POST-MASTECTOMY RECONSTRUCTION: WHEN?

Immediate breast reconstruction produces high satisfaction rates in women undergoing prophylactic mastectomy,[1] and more cancer patients are now offered an immediate reconstruction in an attempt to alleviate some of the psychological trauma from loss of the breast. After a more extensive surgical procedure, however, the incidence of complications is higher. Patients may have the unrealistic expectation that the reconstructed breast will be an exact replica of the original. Complications with healing may force a delay in the start of adjuvant therapy and, in the longer term, cosmetic results may be affected by the need for radiotherapy, so that there are some arguments for delayed reconstruction.

Key points 1

- Immediate breast reconstruction produces high satisfaction rates in women undergoing prophylactic mastectomy.

Christopher Khoo FRCS
Consultant Plastic Surgeon, The Bridge Clinic, Maidenhead, Berkshire SL6 8DG, UK.
E-mail: ctkkhoo@bakersbarn.net

SKIN-SPARING MASTECTOMY

The preservation of the skin envelope in 'skin-sparing mastectomy' allows immediate restoration of breast volume, either using a submuscular expander/implant, or an autogenous tissue flap reconstruction. In a series of 106 skin sparing mastectomies, reconstruction with a muscle sparing TRAM flap or DIEP flap, consistently produced good aesthetic results.[2]

PARTIAL BREAST DEFECTS

Randomised trials have shown that wide local excision or subcutaneous mastectomy and nodal irradiation provide the same degree of local control for cancers detected at an early stage, and survival rates following adequate local resection are similar to those obtained after modified radical mastectomy. These observations have stimulated the development of breast preserving surgery, with immediate reconstruction of the defect, which is not precluded by the need for axillary surgery. Patients who opt for a one-stage procedure should be made aware pre-operatively of the potential need for further surgery if positive margins are reported.[3]

The wide range of partial mastectomy defects following breast conservation therapy creates a challenge to surgical decision making. A management algorithm taking into account the nature and position of the tumour, breast size, the surgical defect, and the timing and extent of radiation has recently been proposed to help in selecting the most appropriate reconstructive procedures.[4]

ONCOPLASTIC SURGERY

The combination of oncological excision with conventional aesthetic breast moulding techniques to reconstruct partial mastectomy defects is known as 'oncoplastic surgery' or 'therapeutic mammoplasty'. Clinicopathological factors determine the type of reconstruction which can be offered and these include cancer stage, type, prior or planned radiation therapy or chemotherapy, and axillary sentinel node status.[5] Patients' preferences, the availability of donor tissue, the volume and shape of the contra-lateral breast, pre-existing scars, and heavy smoking which may compromise flap viability all require consideration.

Breast conservation may replace mastectomy in many patients, avoiding total breast reconstruction and producing better cosmetic results.

Key points 2

- The combination of oncological excision with aesthetic breast moulding techniques conserves breast tissue and avoids the need for mastectomy in many patients.

THE LATISSIMUS DORSI MUSCULOCUTANEOUS FLAP AND VARIANTS

The latissimus dorsi musculocutaneous flap has been a mainstay of autogenous tissue reconstruction, either as pedicled or free flap with microsurgical anastomoses.

The branching intramuscular blood supply allows the use of a pedicled latissimus dorsi 'miniflap' to be split from the muscle to replace up to a quarter of breast volume. Adequate resection can be achieved whilst avoiding deformity. An 'extended' latissimus dorsi flap, including additional adjacent fat, is an alternative to abdominal tissue procedures in patients who are not suitable for more extensive procedures. The extra volume may avoid the need for an implant. However, there will be a longer scar on the back and less tissue bulk is available when compared with more generous donor sites, such as the abdomen.

LATISSIMUS DORSI FLAP MORBIDITY

In a recent study of shoulder morbidity and recovery after latissimus dorsi breast reconstruction, it was found that range of motion, strength, function and pain were still abnormal 6 months after surgery, but had normalised by 1 year.[6] Patients undergoing reconstruction with an extended latissimus dorsi flap had poorer recovery than a latissimus flap with an implant.

Seromas of the donor site are common, but their incidence may be reduced by quilting sutures to eliminate dead space, or the use of steroids.[7]

MUSCULOCUTANEOUS FLAPS: THE TRANSVERSE UPPER GRACILIS (TUG) FLAP

In women with smaller breasts, the transverse upper gracilis (TUG) flap provides adequate tissue for reconstruction. Based on the ascending branch of the medial circumflex femoral artery, it provides a skin paddle of 25 cm × 10 cm, and avoids donor site scars on the back, the abdomen, or the buttock area. Closure of the donor site provides a thigh lift.[8]

ABDOMINAL FLAPS

A number of abdominal flaps have been developed since the description of the original musculocutaneous transverse rectus abdominis flap. The same area of abdominal skin and subcutaneous fat are raised, but with a muscle-sparing (MS) progression from inclusion of the entire rectus abdominis muscle (MS-0), preservation of the lateral segment (MS-1), the lateral and medial segments (MS-2), or sparing the entire muscle (MS-3) as in a perforator flap raised on a deep inferior epigastric (DIEP) perforating vessel. It has also been proposed that the muscle-sparing classification should specify whether it is the medial (MS 1-M) or lateral segment of the rectus muscle (MS1-L) that has been spared, as the motor innervation enters from the lateral side.[9]

The superficial inferior epigastric artery (SIEA) arises from the common femoral or superficial circumflex vessels, so the pedicle of a flap can be raised without violating the fascia as it arises superficial to the rectus sheath.

PERFORATOR FLAPS: THE ABDOMEN

Soft tissue flaps based on perforator vessels spare donor site muscle. Microsurgical expertise, confidence in dealing with anatomical variations, and clinical judgement in choosing the most appropriate flap donor site are essential for consistent outcomes.[10]

The deep inferior epigastric artery perforator (DIEP) flap is established as a preferred breast reconstructive option.

Whilst initial priorities related to flap viability, there has been increasing concern about the preservation of donor site integrity. The motor nerves to the rectus abdominis muscle enter its posterior surface and run with the lateral row perforators and are at risk during the raising of a DIEP flap. The medial row perforators are not related to motor nerves, and these are now recommended for inclusion when the flap is raised to preserve abdominal muscle function.[11]

GLUTEAL PERFORATOR FLAPS

Superior and inferior gluteal artery perforator flaps (S-GAP and I-GAP) depend on a pedicle which is dissected free of donor site muscle, giving increased length, avoiding the need for vein grafts in the recipient site and reducing donor site morbidity arising from muscle loss or adjacent nerve damage.[12]

ABDOMINAL FLAP DONOR SITE COMPLICATIONS

The free TRAM, DIEP and SIEA flaps have advantages and disadvantages relative to each other in terms of pedicle length, vessel calibre, and the safe area of soft tissue vascularity.

TRAM flaps are reliable. In a longitudinal series of 569 free rectus abdominis musculocutaneous flaps on 500 consecutive patients over a 12-year period, there were recoverable thrombotic complications in 6% of patients and only one total flap loss, an overall success rate of 99.7%.[13]

In terms of donor site complications, one study compared 72 consecutive superficial inferior epigastric (SIEA) flaps with the series of 569 consecutive muscle sparing free TRAM flaps cited above;[13] it was found that the SIEA flap had a lower rate of hernia and bulging, but a higher rate of thrombotic complications with a total flap loss rate of 2.9% versus 0.3%. The authors concluded that careful consideration should be given before SIEA flap reconstruction is undertaken.[14] These conclusions are contradicted in another study of 179 patients undergoing breast reconstruction with SIEA, DIEP and muscle-sparing TRAM flaps when morbidity was lowest with SIEA flaps,[15] suggesting that patient selection and surgical expertise remain major factors in achieving satisfactory outcomes.

THE PLACE OF IMPLANT RECONSTRUCTION

The majority of patients who undergo post-mastectomy reconstruction will have a procedure which involves the placement of an implant for restoration of volume, either in a skin-expansion process, or in conjunction with an autogenous flap.

Outcomes were surveyed in a study of 186 consecutive patients who underwent immediate breast reconstruction with either expander/implants, a latissimus dorsi flap, or a TRAM flap. High satisfaction rates were seen across all three reconstructive groups, but the highest patient satisfaction levels were seen in expander/implant reconstructions, despite higher re-operation rates and lower aesthetic scores from four blinded reviewers.[16] An implant reconstruction, where practicable and acceptable to the patient, is the simplest reconstructive technique, and may enable service providers to meet treatment targets better. As with all reconstructive techniques, patients should be aware of the possible need for further procedures and specific implant-related complications.

Key points 3

- The use of an implant is the simplest surgical technique for reconstruction of the breast and produces high patient satisfaction.

COSMETIC BREAST SURGERY

BREAST AUGMENTATION AND CANCER INCIDENCE AND DETECTION

Breast augmentation for cosmetic reasons is widely accepted in the US and Europe. Long-term data show no association between the presence of breast implants and increased breast cancer incidence. A cohort of 3486 Swedish women who underwent cosmetic breast implantation between 1965 and 1993 were followed until 2002, through the nation-wide Swedish Cancer Registry. The mean follow-up was 18.4 years, and the longest 37 years. Breast cancer was lower than predicted to occur, demonstrating a reduced risk.[17]

However, as the population of women with breast implants ages, an increasing number will develop breast cancer. The literature on the radiological and tissue diagnosis of breast cancer in women with a history of augmentation mammaplasty has been reviewed.[18] Special techniques exist for adequately visualising breast tissue in the presence of implants, though views may be affected by capsular contracture. The effectiveness of screening mammography to detect impalpable lesions may be impaired, and women with a family history should receive counselling. Diagnostic fine needle aspiration, percutaneous core and vacuum-assisted biopsy can be safely carried out without increased complications, but percutaneous biopsy should be carried out under image guidance.

GYNAECOMASTIA

A number of surgical techniques are available to treat gynaecomastia (suction-assisted or ultrasound-assisted lipoplasty, circumareolar reduction with round block suture, glandular reduction and skin resection), and have been matched with four grades of severity based on the relationship of the nipple areolar complex to the submammary fold.[19] If no submammary fold is present (Grade I), or if the nipple areolar complex is above the submammary fold (Grade II), a skin-sparing procedure such as a subcutaneous mastectomy, or in combination with liposuction, is indicated. Larger patients, with the nipple areolar complex at the level of the submammary fold (Grade III) will need a periolar reduction adenectomy with liposuction and skin excision. Grade IV patients require a reduction mastoplasty and possible adjuvant procedures such as lipoplasty and scar revision.

GIGANTOMASTIA

The reduction of over 1.5 kg of tissue per breast has been loosely accepted as the common denominator of this condition, but a new classification based on cause, management and prognosis is proposed as being more clinically relevant to patient management. Following a meta-analysis of all published cases, three groups have been described:[20]

Group I   Idiopathic, spontaneous breast growth;

Group II   Excessive breast growth related to endogenous hormone imbalance; and

Group III Excessive breast growth induced by a pharmacological agent.

Group I patients respond well to breast reduction. Group II patients who suffer aggressive and unremitting breast growth may require mastectomy, with or without breast reconstruction. Group III patients often respond to cessation of drug therapy, but surgery may also be necessary.

FACIAL RECONSTRUCTION

CLINICAL EXPERIENCE: PARTIAL FACE TRANSPLANTATION

A scalp and two-ear transplant was performed on a 72-year-old woman in Nanjing, China in 2003. Four partial face transplants have now been undertaken by composite tissue allografts (CTAs): the first in France in November 2005 for traumatic loss of the mid face of a 38-year-old woman; the second in China in April 2006 to replace the nose, cheek and lips of a 30-year-old man mauled by a bear; and the third in France in January 2007 to replace the nose, mouth, chin, and part of the cheeks of a 29-year-old man severely disfigured by neurofibromatosis.[21] He underwent a graft of the lower two-thirds of the face revascularised from a single facial pedicle. The transferred tissue included the perioral muscles, the facial nerves (VII, V2 and V3) and the parotid glands.[22]

A fourth transplant of 80% of the face is reported to have taken place in Cleveland, Ohio, USA in December 2008. The nose, sinuses, and part of the upper jaw were included in an extensive post-traumatic reconstruction in a female patient.

ANATOMICAL BASIS: SOFT TISSUE TRANSFER

Technical aspects of full-face harvesting have been explored in cadaver studies in an attempt to expedite donor tissue transfer and reduce warm ischaemia times. Paired superficial musculo-aponeurotic system (SMAS) plane composite facial-scalp flaps were harvested on either a superficial temporal or facial artery pedicle, or on the external carotid artery. The former technique was half as long (mean, 113 ± 6 min) and offered good perfusion whilst avoiding potential damage within the carotid and submental triangles.[23]

FULL-FACE TRANSPLANTATION: THE FUTURE?

Complete osteocutaneous face transplantation, (transplantation of the maxillofacial skeleton with overlying soft tissues) has not been clinically performed. Cadaver studies have now been undertaken to assess the feasibility of this technique. Using subperiosteal harvest of the soft tissues, including a LeFort III bony segment, osteosynthesis allowed secure fixation and an exact soft tissue fit after customisation of the graft to its recipient site. Portions of the nasal septum and the ethmoid were trimmed, and bony gaps at the zygomatic arches were filled with interpositional bone grafts. Many technical challenges remain but osteocutaneous replacement offers the hope of restoration for the most severe facial defects.[24]

Key points 4

- No patient has yet undergone replacement of the entire face. Technical challenges with surgery are being met, but there are continuing concerns relating to long-term immunosuppression and the ethical and psychological consequences of failure.

IMMUNOSUPPRESSION

Experience with composite tissue allotransplantation now includes skin, solid organs, nerves, tendons, bones, joints and single and double hands. Abdominal wall muscle, tongue and uterus have also been transplanted. Immunotherapy approaches include induction, maintenance and rescue therapy for episodes of rejection, and immunosuppressive agents themselves may be the cause of toxicity or permit infective episodes, and cardiovascular, renal and diabetic co-morbidity.[25]

Despite the high antigenicity of the skin, there is hope that novel agents, topical immunosuppressant application, and strategies to induce tolerance may result in reduced clinical risk.

FACIAL RECONSTRUCTION WITH CONVENTIONAL TECHNIQUES

Expanded flaps

Conservative surgeons point out that there are established techniques for autogenous tissue reconstruction which avoid the need for life-time immunosuppression. A pedicled expanded transposition flap from the shoulder has been used extensively for facial reconstruction. Facial aesthetic units are respected, and are broken into areas with minimal definition and structure, and central units with a high degree of contour definition. High definition areas require reconstruction of the infrastructure, and the algorithm provides for tissue replacement with flaps, composite grafts and full thickness or partial thickness grafts. This integrated approach makes use of surgical 'skill, patience and courage' to achieve favourable aesthetic results.[26]

Free flaps

Using microsurgical free tissue transfer, a thin bipedicled groin flap measuring 30 cm × 11 cm, vascularised on both sides by the superficial circumflex iliac arteries, maintains enhanced vascularity allowing the thinning of the central portion of the flap. This area, on the anterior neck, is within a well perfused area and can be thinned to achieve good neck definition in reconstruction of the face and chin.[27]

When conventional local tissue, such as a forehead flap, is precluded from use (*e.g.* after burn damage), complete nasal loss can be restored using free tissue transfer. Composite osteocutaneous tissue flaps are too bulky to achieve fine definition but the use of a thin flap, such as the radial forearm flap can be used in a soft tissue sandwich, with local tissue being turned down to line the nose and a cantilever bone graft being sandwiched between layers of vascular tissue to restore the nasal bridge.[28]

WOUND HEALING AND TISSUE REPAIR

VACUUM-ASSISTED WOUND CLOSURE

The vacuum-assisted closure device, first introduced in 1997, is now widely used for wound management. Suction up to 125 mmHg is applied to the wound through polyurethane foam with a pore size of 400–600 μm, under a semi-occlusive dressing. Granulation tissue formation increases, as does blood velocity, while the wound area reduces as oedema fluid and inflammatory cytokines and other proteins are removed. In an experimental model, full-thickness wounds in diabetic rats were divided into different treatment groups to investigate the separate components of the vacuum-assisted closure device. It was concluded that wounds exposed to polyurethane foam are more vascular because of angiogenesis triggered by the foam, whereas the vacuum itself stimulates cell proliferation.[29]

Key point 5

- The angiogenesis and cell proliferation stimulated by vacuum therapy may be combined with other materials such as cryopreserved dermis or porcine mesh to promote healing and facilitate wound closure.

FAT GRAFTING

The use of autogenous fat for use as a biological filler has become re-established as an accepted technique in reconstructive surgery.[30] When fat transfer was first performed over a century ago, discrete fatty masses (such as lipoma tissue) were used with universally poor outcomes due to re-absorption, volume loss, the development of oil cysts and calcification. Current techniques involve the harvesting of fat using suction techniques.[31] Pre-adipocytes constitute 10% of the cell population, and are responsible for graft survival because of their capacity for proliferation. Preferred donor sites are the abdomen and either the inner or outer thigh, and flank. Small volumes of fat are injected into the recipient site, creating multiple tunnels at different planes and with small volumes of fat in order to minimise ischaemia and encourage revascularisation.

FAT-DERIVED STEM CELLS

Mesenchymal stem cells have pluripotentiality to differentiate into different cell lines, and can be obtained in limited quantities from adult bone marrow or from embryos. Adipose-derived stem cells can be separated from aspirates of fat cells in large volume, and without ethical concerns. They have an intense potential for proliferation, enhance vascularity and promote the preservation of fat cells and increase fat volume with applications in tissue engineering, such as bone reconstruction and post-irradiation skin damage.[32]

Key point 6

- Aspirated fat contains stem cells which have intense potential for proliferation and to enhance vascularity, with positive benefits for wound healing and tissue repair.

CLINICAL INDICATIONS

Fat injections have been used for facial contour correction, as autogenous augmentation for vocal cords, as epidural grafts after lumbar disc surgery, in cranial base defects, and for augmenting sphincters.

The most common indication is now in breast surgery. Fat injection has been used for correction of deformity after radiotherapy or previous reconstructive surgery, to add volume ('lipo-filling'), to correct contour deformities following flap or implant surgery, or to address radiation changes. It has been used for correction of congenital abnormalities (*e.g.* Poland's syndrome) and cosmetic augmentation.

COMPLICATIONS OF FAT TRANSFER

Reservations about fat transfer techniques in the breast relate partly to loss of volume, but mainly to radiological changes (microcalcifications, fat cysts, and appearances associated with fat necrosis), though it is felt that experience allows these distinctly benign changes to be distinguished from other significant forms of calcification. Outcomes are technique dependent, but it is claimed that that breast shape and softness can be restored with an acceptable level of complications.[33]

TISSUE FLAPS: APPLICATIONS, DESIGN AND MONITORING

CLINICAL APPLICATIONS OF MICROSURGICAL RECONSTRUCTION

Microsurgical techniques have become fully established over the last four decades, allowing confident, safe and successful tissue transfer. In the challenging context of paediatric reconstructions, experience has been reported with 433 transfers over 29 years with a 99.8% success rate and with only 9% complications, most of which were salvaged. Defects across the entire body were repaired and, despite greater technical difficulties in children in comparison with adults, it was concluded that free tissue transfers in children are safer because they are generally more healthy.[34]

THE UPPER LIMB

Reconstruction of the upper extremity may be achieved with pedicled and free radial forearm flaps or reverse-pedicled upper arm flap which can cover the elbow. Extensive excisions for malignant disease which would previously have led to amputation have been successfully reconstructed primarily with microsurgical osteocutaneous transfer of a vascularised fibular flap to the arm. Confident understanding of patterns of vascularisation at a very distal level have allowed the creation of very thin tailored flaps where tissue has been sculpted ('microdissected') without damage to vascular perfusion, and allowing aesthetic reconstruction by preservation of perforators for upper limb reconstruction.[35]

THE LOWER LIMB

Since 1984, the anterolateral thigh flap has been used extensively for soft tissue reconstruction in the upper extremity and the head and neck, by free microsurgical transfer. Now, the simple local transfer of a large skin island of up to 15 cm × 15 cm with a long vascular pedicle has allowed straightforward reconstruction of the internal pelvis, lateral thigh, and groin and genitoperineal areas. The flap can be designed to be musculocutaneous (with a portion of vastus lateralis muscle), or as a perforator flap taking only skin.[36] The concept of 'free style flap harvest' is based on the localisation of a feeding perforator vessel as it enters an area of fascia and skin overlying muscle bellies and intermuscular septa. After Doppler localisation of the vessel, dissection proceeds at subfascial level to raise a flap which is geometrically designed to be able to move to cover a defect. The perforator vessel is the pivot point and only attachment, and this allows the rotation of the flap up to 180°, similar to the two blades of a propeller. Part of the donor site defect is covered by the flap and the remaining area is skin grafted.[37]

Earlier combined orthopaedic and plastic surgery guidelines for the management of complex tibial fractures[38] are now in the process of extensive revision. Current best practice relating to primary emergency treatment in specialist centres; proposals for accurate, simple and reproducible classification of injuries; the principles of wound management, including debridement, decontamination and preservation of bone; degloving, compartment syndrome and vascular in juries; the management of open fractures, and soft tissue reconstruction have all been considered. The management of bone and soft tissue complications, guidelines for amputation, outcome measures, and the specific care of paediatric fractures are covered in the revised guidelines, to be issued in 2009.

FLAP DESIGN

Duplex scanners display grey-scale images in real time, and colour Doppler scanners add colour onto the grey image and display blood velocity, which are useful pre-operatively. The success of perforator flaps is enhanced by such techniques which show the vessels *in situ* before the pedicle is dissected. However, in a series of 31 free thoracodorsal artery perforator free flaps, a sterile Doppler probe was used intra-operatively to define perforators as the flaps were raised, with the subsequent loss of only one flap.[39]

POSTOPERATIVE MONITORING

Near-infrared spectroscopy has been shown to be a reliable non-invasive method for monitoring blood circulation in cutaneous flaps and is also effective in monitoring buried flaps, such as fibular flaps.[40] Dependable postoperative monitoring is also provided by the use of an implantable 20-MHz Doppler probe consisting of an electrode and a cuff, which allows direct and continuous vessel monitoring of the anastomoses. The probe may be used as the sole postoperative monitoring device and is removed when the flap is stable.[41]

Key point 7

- Doppler probes can be used pre-operatively or intra-operatively to define vessels and measure blood flow. Implantable Doppler probes can also be used for postoperative flap monitoring.

Key points for clinical practice

- Immediate breast reconstruction produces high satisfaction rates in women undergoing prophylactic mastectomy.

- The combination of oncological excision with aesthetic breast moulding techniques conserves breast tissue and avoids the need for mastectomy in many patients.

- The use of an implant is the simplest surgical technique for reconstruction of the breast and produces high patient satisfaction.

(continued)

Key points for clinical practice *(continued)*

- No patient has yet undergone replacement of the entire face. Technical challenges with surgery are being met, but there are continuing concerns relating to long-term immunosuppression and the ethical and psychological consequences of failure.

- The angiogenesis and cell proliferation stimulated by vacuum therapy may be combined with other materials such as cryopreserved dermis or porcine mesh to promote healing and facilitate wound closure.

- Aspirated fat contains stem cells which have intense potential for proliferation and to enhance vascularity, with positive benefits for wound healing and tissue repair.

- Doppler probes can be used pre-operatively or intra-operatively to define vessels and measure blood flow. Implantable Doppler probes can also be used for postoperative flap monitoring.

References

1. Isern AE, Tengrup I, Loman N *et al.* Aesthetic outcome, patient satisfaction, and health-related quality of life in women at high risk undergoing prophylactic mastectomy and immediate breast reconstruction. *J Plast Reconstr Aesthet Surg* 2008; **61**: 1177–1187.
2. Scholz T, Kretsis V, Kobayashi MR, Evans GR. Long-term outcomes after primary breast reconstruction using a vertical skin pattern for skin-sparing mastectomy. *Plast Reconstr Surg* 2008; **122**: 1603–1611.
3. The Association of Breast Surgery at the British Association of Surgical Oncology, and The British Association of Plastic Aesthetic and Reconstructive Surgeons. Oncoplastic breast surgery – A guide to good practice. *Eur J Surg Oncol* 2007; **33**: S1–S23.
4. Kronowitz SJ, Kuerer, HM, Buchholz TA, Valero V, Hunt KK. A management algorithm and practical oncoplastic surgical techniques for repairing partial mastectomy defects. *Plast Reconstr Surg* 2008; **122**: 1631–1647.
5. McCulley S, Macmillan R. Planning and use of therapeutic mammaplasty – Nottingham approach. *Br J Plast Surg* 2005; **58**: 889–901.
6. Glassey NM, Perks GB, McCulley SJ. A prospective assessment of shoulder morbidity and recovery time scales following latissimus dorsi breast reconstruction. *Plast Reconstr Surg* 2008; **122**: 1334–1340.
7. Taghizadeh R, Shoaib T, Hart AM *et al.* Triamcinolone reduces seroma re-accumulation in the extended latissimus dorsi donor site. *J Plast Reconstr Aesthet Surg* 2008; **61**: 636–642.
8. Arnez ZN, Pogorelec D, Planinsek F, Ahcan U. Breast reconstruction by the free transverse gracilis (TUG) flap. *Br J Plast Surg* 2004; **57**: 20–26.
9. Bajaj AK, Chevray PM, Chang DW. Comparison of donor site complications and functional outcomes in free muscle sparing TRAM flap and free DIEP breast reconstruction. *Plast Reconstr Surg* 2006; **117**: 737–746.
10. Blondeel PN, Morris SF, Hallock GG *et al.* (eds) *Perforator Flaps: anatomy, technique and clinical applications*, vols I and II. St Louis, MO: Quality Medical Publishing, 2006; 37.
11. Rozen WM, Ashton MW, Murray ACA, Taylor GI. Avoiding denervation of rectus abdominis in DIEP flap harvest: the importance of medial row perforators. *Plast Reconstr Surg* 2008; **122**: 710–716.
12. Heitman C, Levine JL, Allen RJ. Gluteal artery perforator flaps. *Clin Plast Surg* 2007; **34**: 123–130.

13. Vega S, Smartt JM, Jiang S *et al*. 500 consecutive patients with free TRAM flap breast reconstruction: a single surgeon's experience. *Plast Reconstr Surg* 2008; **122**: 329–339.
14. Selber JC, Samra F, Bristol M *et al*. A head-to-head comparison between the muscle-sparing free TRAM and the SIEA flaps: is the rate of flap loss worth the gain in abdominal wall function? *Plast Reconstr Surg* 2008; **122**: 348–355.
15. Wu LC, Bajaj A, Chang DW *et al*. Comparison of donor site morbidity of SIEA, DIEP and muscle-sparing TRAM flaps for breast reconstruction. *Plast Reconstr Surg* 2008; **122**: 702–709.
16. Spear SL, Newman MK, Bedford MS *et al*. A retrospective analysis of outcomes using three common methods for immediate breast reconstruction. *Plast Reconstr Surg* 2008; **122**: 340–347.
17. McLaughlin JK, Lipworth L, Fryzek JP *et al*. Long-term cancer risk among Swedish women with cosmetic breast implants: an update of a nationwide study. *J Natl Cancer Inst* 2006; **98**: 557–560.
18. McIntosh SA, Horgan K. Augmentation mammaplasty: effect on diagnosis of breast cancer. *J Plast Reconstr Aesthet Surg* 2008; **61**: 124–129.
19. Cordova A, Moschella F. Algorithm for clinical evaluation and surgical treatment of gynaecomastia. *J Plast Reconstr Aesthet Surg* 2008; **61**: 41–49.
20. Dancey A, Khan M, Dawson J, Peart F. Gigantomastia – a classification and review of the literature. *J Plast Reconstr Aesthet Surg* 2008; **61**: 493–502.
21. Dubernard J-M, Devauchelle B. Face transplantation. *Lancet* 2008; **372**: 603–604.
22. Meningaud J-P, Paraskevas A, Ingallina F, Bouhana E, Lantieri L. Face transplant graft procurement: a preclinical and clinical study. *Plast Reconstr Surg* 2008; **122**: 1383–1389.
23. Wang HY, Li QF, Zheng SW *et al*. Cadaveric comparison of two facial flap-harvesting techniques for alloplastic facial transplantation. *J Plast Reconstr Aesthet Surg* 2007; **60**: 1175–1181.
24. Follmar KE, Baccarani A, Das RR *et al*. Osteocutaneous face transplantation. *J Plast Reconstr Aesthet Surg* 2008; **61**: 518–524.
25. Whitaker IS, Duggan EM, Alloway RR *et al*. Composite tissue allotransplantation: a review of relevant immunological issues for plastic surgeons. *J Plast Reconstr Aesthet Surg* 2008; **61**: 481–492.
26. Spence RJ. An algorithm for total and subtotal facial reconstruction using an expanded transposition flap: a 20-year experience. *Plast Reconstr Surg* 2008; **121**: 795–805.
27. Matsumine H, Sakurai H, Nakajima Y *et al*. Use of a bipedicled thin groin flap in reconstruction of postburn anterior neck contracture. *Plast Reconstr Surg* 2008; **122**: 782–785.
28. Sinha M, Scott JR, Watson SB. Prelaminated free radial forearm flap for a total nasal reconstruction. *J Plast Reconstr Aesthet Surg* 2008; **61**: 953–957.
29. Scherer SS, Pietromaggiori G, Mathews JC *et al*. The mechanism of action of the vacuum-assisted closure device. *Plast Reconstr Surg* 2008; **122**: 786–797.
30. Chan CW, McCulley SJ, Macmillan RD. Autologous fat transfer – a review of the literature with a focus on breast cancer surgery. *J Plast Reconstr Aesthet Surg* 2008; **61**: 1438–1448.
31. Pu LLQ, Coleman SR, Cui X, Fergusion REH, Vasconez HC. Autologous fat grafts harvested and refined by the Coleman technique: a comparative study. *Plast Reconstr Surg* 2008; **122**: 932–937.
32. Rigotti G, Marchi A, Galie M *et al*. Clinical treatment of radiotherapy tissue damage by lipoaspirate transplant: a healing process mediated by adipose-derived adult stem cells. *Plast Reconstr Surg* 2007; **119**: 1409–1422.
33. Delay E, Gosset J, Toussoun G, Delaporte T, Delbaere M. Efficacy of lipomodelling for the management of sequelae of breast cancer conservative treatment. *Ann Chir Plast Esthét* 2008; **53**: 153–168.
34. Upton J, Guo L. Paediatric free tissue transfer: a 29-year experience with 433 transfers. *Plast Reconstr Surg* 2008; **121**: 1725–1737.
35. Kimura N, Saito M, Sumiya Y, Itoh N. Reconstruction of hand skin defects by microdissected mini anterolateral thigh perforator flaps. *J Plast Reconstr Aesthet Surg* 2008; **61**: 1073–1077.
36. Ng RWM, Chan J YW, Mok V, Li GKH. Clinical use of a pedicled anterolateral thigh flap.

J Plast Reconstr Aesthet Surg 2008; **61**: 158–164.

37. Pignatti M, Pasqualini MN, Governa M, Bruti M, Rigotti G. Propeller flaps for leg reconstruction. *J Plast Reconstr Aesthet Surg* 2008; **61**: 777–783.

38. A report by the British Orthopaedic Association/British Association of Plastic Surgeons Working Party on the management of open tibial fractures. September 1997. *Br J Plast Surg* 1997; **50**: 570–583.

39. Lee SH, Mun GH. Transverse thoracodorsal artery perforator flaps: experience with 31 free flaps. *J Plast Reconstr Aesthet Surg* 2008; **61**: 372–379.

40. Cai Z, Zhang J, Zhang J *et al.* Evaluation of near infrared spectroscopy in monitoring postoperative regional tissue oxygen saturation for fibular flaps. *J Plast Reconstr Aesthet Surg* 2008; **61**: 289–296.

41. Smit JM, Zeebregts CJ, Acosta R. Timing of presentation of the first signs of vascular compromise dictates the salvage outcome of free flap transfers. *Plast Reconstr Surg* 2008; **122**: 991–992.

Joanna Franks Irving Taylor

16

Randomised clinical trials in surgery 2008

This chapter reviews a selection of randomised clinical trials, published in 2008, which relate to general surgical issues. Well-designed, randomised, controlled trials aim to provide a platform of robust evidence on which surgical management can be built. A number of good quality meta-analyses have also been included as they provide additional evidence to aid clinical practice. The aim is to highlight areas which may influence clinical practice and future patient management.

HEAD AND NECK

The efficacy of tranexamic acid on the duration of drainage after head and neck surgery was assessed in a randomised controlled trial.[1] Vacuum drains are frequently used after head and neck surgery to reduce the formation of either haematomas or seromas and reduce pressure on approximated skin flaps. However, prolonged drain placement increases the risk of wound infection[2] as well as hospital stay. The 26 patients in the study arm of the trial received a pre-operative dose of tranexamic acid (intravascular 10 mg/kg) followed by a continuous infusion (1 mg/kg/h) during the operation. The 29 patients in the control group followed the same protocol but received normal saline. There was a significant difference in the volume drained by both groups, an average of 49.7 ml in the study arm compared with 88.8 ml in the control arm ($P = 0.041$). However, no significant difference in the duration of

Joanna Franks MBBS(Hons) BSc(Hons) MRCS MSc (for correspondence)
Specialist Registrar in General Surgery, Division of Surgery and Interventional Science, University College London, 74 Huntley Street, London WC1E 6AU, UK. E-mail: drjlfranks@aol.com

Irving Taylor MD ChM FMedSci FRCPS(Glas) FHEA
Professor of Surgery, Director of Medical Studies and Vice Dean UCL Medical School, University College London, 74 Huntley Street, London WC1E 6AU, UK. E-mail: irving.taylor@ucl.ac.uk

drainage was found, 2.69 days and 3.07 days for the study and control patients, respectively. The authors of this study concluded that there is no advantage to the use of prophylactic tranexamic acid in this setting. Unfortunately, the study did not include patients who have undergone previous radiotherapy. This cohort of patients are more likely to develop postoperative haematomas; therefore, the demonstration of a significant reduction in drain duration might have made the greatest impact on practical management.

Key point 1

- Tranexamic acid can be used to reduce the volume drained after head and neck surgery.

PILONIDAL SINUS

Pilonidal sinus is a common condition seen regularly in general surgical out-patients. Despite this, the management of pilonidal disease remains a contentious issue. Several surgical alternatives exist from simple excision combined with open healing to primary closure. Advocates of primary closure favour different methods but can be broadly divided into methods which are either midline (closure lies in the midline of the natal cleft) or off-midline, lying outside the natal cleft.

A recently published systematic review and meta-analyses of randomised, controlled trials[3] aimed to determine the relative effects of these different management approaches. The pooled results demonstrate that wounds heal more quickly after primary closure, as demonstrated by a faster return to work, than when left to heal by secondary intention. There was no significant difference in the rate of surgical site infection between primary and secondary closure. However, primary closure carries an increased risk of recurrence. The data available equate to recurrence rates of 14 patients per 100 undergoing primary closure compared to 5 per 100 undergoing open healing. When considering the data relating to primary closure, the off-midline methods show a clear benefit compared with midline closure. The recurrence rates for off-midline closure were significantly lower (1.4%) than with midline closure (10.3%). In addition, off-midline closure recorded fewer infections and quicker wound healing.

Key point 2

- In the management of pilonidal disease, treatment method should be based on patient and surgeon preference with consideration of the patients' goals for therapy. Off-midline closure shows benefits for most clinical and patient outcomes.

UPPER GI SURGERY

ANTI-REFLUX SURGERY

Two trials, Anvari et al.[4] and Mehta et al.,[5] have demonstrated the superiority of surgery over medical treatment for the management of gastro-oesophageal reflux disease (GORD). Nissen fundoplication (360° wrap) is the standard operation for GORD. Recently, consideration has been given to the recognised postoperative complication of dysphagia. To improve the surgical results, it has been proposed that the anti-reflux surgery should be tailored to individual cases according to their pre-existing oesophageal motility.

The Toupet procedure (270° wrap) has been recommended for patients with pre-existing dysmotility as this cohort of patients are thought more likely to develop postoperative dysphagia. A randomised, controlled trial[6] has evaluated tailored anti-reflux surgery by comparing the Nissen and Toupet fundoplications. A cohort of 200 patients underwent pre-operative assessment including a clinical interview, endoscopy, 24-h pH monitoring and oesophageal manometry. Of these, 100 patients (half with motility disorders and half without) underwent a laparoscopic Nissen procedure or Toupet fundoplication. Postoperative follow-up included a repeat of the pre-operative assessments. After 2 years, 85% of both the Nissen and Toupet patients were satisfied with their operative result. Dysphagia was more frequent following a Nissen fundoplication (19 patients) than after a Toupet (8 patients; $P < 0.05$). This did not correlate with individual pre-operative motility results. The Toupet procedure controlled symptoms as well as a Nissen fundoplication.

Key points 3–5

- Tailoring anti-reflux surgery according to oesophageal motility is not indicated.

- Motility disorders are not correlated with postoperative dysphagia.

- The Toupet procedure should be considered when performing anti-reflux surgery as it is able to control symptoms with a lower rate of dysphagia.

PANCREAS

Complications secondary to chronic pancreatitis are common. The optimal choice of technique for the surgical treatment of pancreatic head lesions in chronic pancreatitis has been the subject of a recent systematic review and meta-analysis.[7] Comparing duodenum-preserving pancreatic head resection with a pancreaticoduodenectomy demonstrated no significant difference in postoperative pain relief, overall mortality or morbidity. However, in the short-term, patients who underwent a duodenum-preserving pancreatic head resection had the benefit of reduced intra-operative blood loss, shorter hospital stay, weight gain and improved occupational rehabilitation.

The long-term follow-up of a randomised, controlled trial comparing the surgical approach used for pancreatic head resection in the management of chronic pancreatitis has recently been reported.[8] Forty patients were originally enrolled in this study. Half underwent a duodenum-preserving pancreatic head resection according to Beger, the remainder underwent a pylorus preserving Whipple procedure. Long-term follow-up included mortality, morbidity, pain, quality of life and endocrine and exocrine function at a median follow up of 7 years and 14 years. There were five late deaths in each group. No differences were demonstrated in pain status and exocrine function. The only significant difference in quality of life was loss of appetite in the Whipple group at 14 years. Loss of endocrine function was demonstrated in both groups, by the development of diabetes mellitus, which was diagnosed in 47% of patients who had a Beger procedure and 79% who underwent a Whipple procedure ($P = 0.128$).

Tailored, organ-sparing procedures are believed to be potentially superior to standard resections in the management of inflammatory pancreatic head tumours as they result in greater preservation of endocrine and exocrine function. A study[9] reported on the long-term results of a randomised trial comparing a classical resection (pylorus-preserving Whipple) with an extended drainage (Frey) for chronic pancreatitis. All the patients who participated in the earlier phase of this trial were contacted and completed a quality-of-life assessment questionnaire. In addition, endocrine function was measured with an oral glucose tolerance test and exocrine function with a faecal chymotrypsin test. The results over a median of 7 years' follow-up showed that both approaches to the treatment of chronic pancreatitis provide adequate pain relief and quality-of-life scores with no difference in endocrine or exocrine function.

Pancreatic cancer is the fourth leading cause of cancer death in men and the fifth in women. Despite this high incidence, the surgical approach to peri-ampullary and pancreatic cancer remains a debated subject. A Cochrane systematic review[10] addressed this question. The study included all published and unpublished, randomised, controlled trials comparing a pancreatico-duodenectomy (classic Whipple) with a pylorus-preserving pancreatico-duodenectomy (pylorus-preserving Whipple). Overall in-hospital mortality, overall survival and morbidity showed no significant difference. Mean operating time and intra-operative blood loss were significantly reduced in the pylorus-preserving Whipple group.

As discussed, partial pancreaticoduodenectomy is the surgical management for various benign and malignant pancreatic disorders. The recognised postoperative complications of a pancreaticoduodenectomy include postoperative pancreatic fistula and delayed gastric emptying. Prophylactic octreotide has been advocated for the prevention of pancreatic fistula formation; however, somatostatin and its analogues have been associated with delayed gastric emptying. A randomised, controlled trial[11] looked at the effect of prophylactic octreotide, by comparing it with normal saline, in patients who underwent pancreaticoduodenectomy. The primary end-point was the incidence of delayed gastric emptying measured by clinical signs, gastric scintigraphy and the hydrogen breath test. Delayed gastric emptying, defined as the need for nasogastric decompression for more than 10 days and/or intolerance of normal diet until the 14th postoperative day was similar between both groups (approximately 20%). Scintigraphy indicated that 34% of the octreotide group and 31% of the control group had delayed gastric emptying at the 7th postoperative day. The hydrogen breath test was maximal after 65.0 ± 6.5 min in the octreotide group compared to 67.0 ± 5.7 min in the control group. Delayed gastric emptying was associated with a significantly longer stay in the intensive care unit, a higher requirement of blood and blood products and secondary antibiotic treatment. Postoperative fistula formation was not reduced in the octreotide group. Secondary findings included pre-operative biliary stenting, which reduced delayed gastric emptying, whereas postoperative bleeding and infection were independent risk factors.

The findings demonstrated by this trial were borne out by a meta-analysis of randomised, controlled trials[12] which concluded that the use of somatostatin and its analogues does not significantly reduce postoperative complications after pancreaticoduodenectomy.

Key points 6–9

- Early advantages of duodenum-preserving pancreatic head resection over a pylorus preserving Whipple in the surgical management of chronic pancreatitis have been demonstrated. These are no longer present after long-term follow-up of up to 14 years.

- Tailored organ preserving drainage of inflammatory masses secondary to chronic pancreatitis has short-term advantages. In the long-term, the results are comparable to surgical resection.

- There is currently no evidence of relevant differences in mortality, morbidity and survival between pylorus-preserving Whipple and classic Whipple in the treatment of peri-ampullary and pancreatic carcinoma.

- In 20% of cases, pancreaticoduodenectomy may be complicated by delayed gastric emptying. The prophylactic use of somato-statin or its analogues has no influence on gastric emptying and does not decrease the incidence of pancreatic fistula.

LAPAROSCOPIC CHOLECYSTECTOMY

The place of laparoscopic surgery for elective cholecystectomy has been firmly established in general surgery. Two randomised trials have been published this year which suggest small modifications to surgical technique that may have significant impact on the patients' experience. Although postoperative pain after a laparoscopic cholecystectomy is less than after an open procedure, shoulder and abdominal discomfort can cause considerable distress. One randomised, controlled trial[13] looked at the effect of intraperitoneal irrigation over the diaphragmatic surface and gallbladder fossa on pain control. A total of 200 patients were divided equally into four groups who received no irrigation, normal saline, lignocaine or bupivicaine irrigation. Visual analogue and verbal rating pain scores were recorded as well as analgesia requirements, vital signs and blood glucose. Patients in the treatment groups showed a significant difference in pain rating scores and analgesia requirements when compared to the control patients. Lignocaine was the most efficacious of the local anaesthetics and had a safe profile when used at the recommended dose.

Another randomised trial[14] looked at umbilical port-site infections. These are associated with complications ranging from inflammation, to dehiscence of the umbilical skin sutures and incisional hernias. Patients with uncomplicated cholelithiasis were randomised into those treated with topical rifamycin and those who were not. Patients were followed up for 60 postoperative days. Topical administration of rifamycin to the umbilicus in the pre-, intra- and postoperative periods was safe, rapid and economic and resulted in a significant reduction in infective complications.

The timing of the laparoscopic approach for the treatment of acute cholecystitis is still the subject of much debate. Several studies comparing early with delayed surgery or reporting on conservative treatment of acute cholecystitis have shown that up to 36% of patients will have recurrent episodes or another gallstone-related complication. A meta-analysis of randomised, clinical trials[15] has been published this year which aimed to determine the best practice in terms of clinical benefit. A total of four studies containing 375 patients were included. The combined results suggest that early cholecystectomy is associated with a reduced total hospital stay. In addition, the patients do not have the inconvenience of two admissions. Surgery in the acute setting does, however, have a significantly longer operating time and postoperative stay. The technical difficulty of laparoscopic cholecystectomy in early cholecystitis with increased complication rates has previously been cited as justification for delayed cholecystectomy. This meta-analysis demonstrated no difference in complications, conversions or postoperative morbidity between patients managed surgically during their acute admission and those who underwent an interval laparoscopic cholecystectomy.

Key points 10–12

- Irrigation of the gallbladder fossa and diaphragmatic surfaces at the end of a laparoscopic cholecystectomy will reduce postoperative pain and analgesic requirements. Irrigation with lignocaine has been shown to be both safe and effective.

- Topical administration of rifamycin to the umbilical port-site is a cost-effective and safe way of reducing localised infection and subsequent sequelae.

- There is likely to be no advantage to initial conservative management and delayed laparoscopic surgery for acute cholecystitis. Laparoscopic cholecystectomy should be considered during the acute admission of all patients suitable for surgery.

VASCULAR

CAROTID ANGIOPLASTY AND STENTING

The role of carotid endarterectomy (CEA) in the treatment of patients with symptomatic and asymptomatic carotid disease is based on the results of five highly regarded, randomised, clinical trials. Since these trials were published, carotid angioplasty with stenting (CAS) has emerged as an alternative option in the management of these patients. Intuitively, endovascular techniques should have clinical advantages over the traditional management of carotid disease. The data from early reports and randomised controlled trials have been reviewed.[16] Early non-randomised results of CAS showed variable results leading to no fewer than eight randomised controlled trials.[17] Meta-analysis of these results is complicated as several trials pre-date the development of cerebral protection devices and the incorporation of dual anti-platelet therapy into their protocols. In addition, four of the symptomatic angioplasty trials were stopped prematurely, three due to excess risk after CAS and one because of funding issues. Results from two recently published trials are now available. In the Stent-Protected Angioplasty versus Carotid Endarterectomy trial (SPACE),[18] the complication rate of ipsilateral stroke or death at 30 days was 6.8% for CAS versus 6.3% for CEA. The Endarterectomy Versus Stenting in Patients with Symptomatic Severe Carotid Stenosis trial (EVA-3S) demonstrated that the risk of death or stroke at 30 days for endovascular treatment was 9.6%, significantly higher than 3.9% seen in the CEA patients. Although CAS performed with embolic protection devices can be an effective treatment for carotid stenosis, there is currently no evidence that it provides better stroke prevention than CEA. As none of the meta-analyses available to date support performing CAS in 'standard risk' patients, CEA remains the gold standard treatment.

When considering the population of high-risk patients with carotid artery stenosis, one is comparing the results of intervention with best medical treatment. The routine use of polypharmacy and pharmaceutical advances are speculated to have improved the outcome of patients treated conservatively; therefore, we must not neglect the fact that the data, on which best medical treatment is based, are now outdated.

The results available thus far suggest that symptomatic patients considered 'high risk' for surgery may be preferentially treated by CAS. Currently, asymptomatic high-risk patients remain the most controversial with no agreement on the most appropriate management strategy. The consensus of opinion is that the development of best medical treatment, timely intervention, interventionalists' experience and analysis of plaque composition may have important influences on future treatment protocols. The results of long-term follow-up and additional trials are awaited; however, the expanded use of CAS outside of randomised trials threatens further studies of alternatives to CEA.

VARICOSE VEINS

Minimally invasive endovenous techniques for varicose veins have been developed and are now challenging conventional saphenofemoral ligation, stripping of the long saphenous vein and multiple phlebectomies of residual varicosities. A recent, randomised, controlled trial[20] has been published which compared the results of endovenous laser ablation (EVLA) with conventional surgery. Consecutive adult patients with primary saphenofemoral incompetence and symptomatic varicose veins were included in the study. All patients had a pre-operative duplex Doppler scan. Patients were randomised to EVLA1 (stepwise laser withdrawal), EVLA2 (continuous laser withdrawal) or surgery. Postoperative results showed that the rate of abolition of reflux in the long saphenous vein and the improvement in the Aberdeen Varicose Vein Symptom Severity Score (AVVSS) were equivalent across treatment groups. However, the return to normal activity was, on average, 5 days earlier with the endovenous treatment with a return to work being recorded on average 13 days sooner than the patients treated by conventional surgery.

One criticism of endovenous treatment has been residual varicosities below the knee, which often require further treatment. This is due, in part, to a reluctance to laser treat the long saphenous vein extensively and is of particular relevance to patients who have been shown pre-operatively to have reflux in the long saphenous vein both above and below the knee. A randomised, controlled trial[21] assessed whether more extensive long saphenous vein ablation enhances varicosity resolution and symptom control. Patients were randomised into three groups – above-knee EVLA, EVLA mid-calf to groin and above-knee EVLA with concomitant below-knee foam sclerotherapy. Compared with standard above-knee EVLA, simultaneous ablation of an incompetent below-knee long saphenous vein resulted in fewer varicosities and superior symptom relief (AVVSS) at 6 weeks. Extended EVLA is, therefore, safe and effective and gives comparable results to foam sclerotherapy.

Key point 13–17

- Carotid endarterectomy (CEA) remains the gold standard treatment for patients with carotid artery stenosis.

- Carotid angioplasty with stenting (CAS) could become the preferred option in symptomatic patients considered high risk for surgery.

- Evidence supporting either CEA or CAS in high-risk asymptomatic patient remains controversial.

- Endovenous laser ablation (EVLA) of varicose veins results in comparable abolition of reflux and improvement in disease-specific quality of life when compared to conventional surgery. The average return to normal activities and work is faster with endovenous treatment.

- EVLA can safely and effectively be used to treat reflux in the long saphenous vein below the knee.

BREAST

Adjuvant therapy is used routinely in the treatment of hormone receptor positive breast cancer. The 2007 St Gallen consensus guidelines recommend ovarian suppression with GnRF analogues in premenopausal women with hormone responsive early breast cancer. The Australian Breast & Colorectal Cancer Study Group Trial-12 (ABCSG-12) was designed to assess the clinical efficacy of goserelin-induced ovarian suppression plus tamoxifen or anastrozole with or without zoledronic acid. A prospective bone-mineral density sub-study was included to quantify the long-term effects of endocrine therapy and concomitant zoledronic acid on bone-mineral density.[22] Goserelin plus tamoxifen or anastrozole for 3 years without simultaneous treatment with zoledronic acid caused significant bone loss of the spine and trochanter. Anastrozole caused greater bone-mineral density loss of the lumber spine than tamoxifen at 36 months. Although there was partial recovery 2 years after completing treatment, patients receiving endocrine treatment alone did not recover their baseline bone-mineral density levels. Those patients who received concomitant zolendronic acid did not suffer from bone loss and measurements of their bone-mineral density showed an improvement at 5 years.

Axillary lymphadenectomy remains an essential part of breast cancer management. The complications of axillary dissection are well known with an estimated rate of seroma formation of 15–81%. An Italian study has been published[23] looking at the effectiveness of fibrin glue in conjunction with collagen patches to reduce seroma formation in level I/II axillary dissection in patients undergoing either a quadrantectomy or mastectomy. All patients were treated with a suction drain which was removed at postoperative day 3 or 4. The patients who were in the treatment arm of the study had a significant reduction in seroma magnitude ($P = 0.004$) and duration ($P = 0.02$) and required fewer evacuative punctures.

Key points 18 and 19

- Ovarian inhibition plus endocrine treatment in premenopausal, hormone-sensitive, breast cancer patients results in significant bone loss. Treatment with anastrozole results in a greater reduction in bone-mineral density than tamoxifen. Concomitant zolendronic acid protects bone-mineral density.

- Use of fibrin glue and collagen patches after axillary lymphadenectomy does not always prevent seroma formation but will reduce seroma magnitude and duration.

References

1. Chen CC, Wang, CC, Wang CP, Lin TH, Lin WD, Liu SA. Prospective, randomized, controlled trial of tranexamic acid in patients who undergo head and neck procedures. *Otolaryngol Head Neck Surg* 2008; **138**: 762–767.
2. Urquhart AC, Berg RL. Neck dissections: predicting postoperative drainage. *Laryngoscope* 2002; **112**: 1294–1298.
3. McCallum IJ, King PM, Bruce J. Healing by primary closure versus open healing after surgery

for pilonidal sinus: systematic review and meta-analysis. *BMJ* 2008; **336**: 868–871.

4. Anavari M, Allen C, Marshall J *et al*. A randomized controlled trial of laparoscopic Nissen fundoplication versus proton pump inhibitors for treatment of patients with chronic gastroeosphageal reflux disease: one-year follow-up. *Surg Innovat* 2006; **13**: 238–249.

5. Mehta S, Bennett J, Mahon D, Rhodes M. Prospective trial of laparoscopic Nissen fundoplication versus proton pump inhibitor therapy for gastroesophageal reflux disease: seven year follow-up. *J Gastrointest Surg* 2006; **10**: 1312–1317.

6. Strate U, Emmermann C, Fibbe C, Layer P, Zornig C. Laparoscopic fundoplication: Nissen versus Toupet two-year outcome of a prospective randomized study of 200 patients regarding pre-operative oesophageal motility. *Surg Endosc* 2008; **22**: 21–30.

7. Diener MK, Rahbari NN, Fischer L *et al*. Duodenum-preserving pancreatic head resection versus pancreatoduodenectomy for surgical treatment of chronic pancreatitis: a systematic review and meta-analysis. *Ann Surg* 2008; **247**: 950–961.

8. Muller MW, Friess H, Martin DJ *et al*. Long-term follow-up of a randomized clinical trial comparing Beger with pylorus-preserving Whipple procedure for chronic pancreatitis. *Br J Surg* 2008; **95**: 350–356.

9. Strate t, Bachmann K, Busch P *et al*. Resection vs drainage in treatment of chronic pancreatitis: long-term results of a randomized trial *Gastroenterology* 2008; **134**: 1406–1411.

10. Diener MK, Heukaufer C, Schwarzer G *et al*. Pancreaticoduodenectomy (classic Whipple) versus pylorus-preserving pancreaticoduodenectomy (pp Whipple) for surgical treatment of periampullary and pancreatic carcinoma. *Cochrane Database Syst Rev* 2008; 16(2): CD006053.

11. Kollmar O, Moussavian M, Richter S *et al*. Prophylactic octreotide and delayed gastric emptying after pancreaticoduodenectomy: results of s prospective randomised double-blinded placebo-controlled trial. *Eur J Surg Oncol* 2008; **34**: 868–875.

12. Zeng Q, Zhang Q, Han S *et al*. Efficacy of somatostatin and its analogues in prevention of postoperative complications after pancreaticoduodenectomy: a meta-analysis of randomized controlled trials. *Pancreas* 2008; **36**: 18–25.

13. Ahmed BH, Ahmed A, Tan D *et al*, Post-laparoscopic cholecystectomy pain: effects of intraperitoneal local anaesthetics on pain control – a randomised prospective double-blinded placebo-controlled trial. *Am Surg* 2008; **74**: 201–209.

14. Neri V, Fersini A, Ambrosi A, Tartaglia N, Valentino TP. Umbilical port-site complications in laparoscopic cholecystectomy: role of topical antibiotic therapy. *J Soc Laparoendosc Surg* 2008; **12**: 126–132.

15. Siddiqui T, MacDonald A, Chong PS, Jenkins IT. Early versus delayed laparoscopic cholecystectomy for acute cholecystitis: a meta-analysis of randomized clinical trials. *Am J Surg* 2008; **195**: 40–47.

16. van der Vaart MG, Meerwaldt R, Reijen M *et al*. Endarterectomy or carotid stenting: the quest continues. *Am J Surg* 2008; **195**: 259–269.

17. Naylor AR. Is surgery still generally the first choice intervention in patients with carotid artery disease? *Surgeon* 2008; **6**: 6–12.

18. Ringleb P, Allenberg J, Bruckmann H *et al*. 30 day results from the SPACE trial of stent-protected angioplasty versus carotid endarterectomy in symptomatic patients: a randomized non-inferiority trial. *Lancet* 2006; **368**: 1239–1247.

19. Mas J, Chatellier G, Beyssen B *et al*. Endarterectomy versus stenting in patients with symptomatic severe carotid stenosis. *N Engl J Med* 2006; **355**: 1660–1671.

20. Darwood R, Theivacumar N, Dellagrammaticas D *et al*. Randomised clinical trial comparing endovenous laser ablation with surgery for the treatment of primary great saphenous varicose veins. *Br J Surg* 2008; **95**: 294–301.

21. Theivacumar N, Dellagrammaticas D, Mavor A, Gough M. Endovenous laser ablation: does standard above-knee great saphenous vein ablation provide optimum results in patients with both above- and below-knee reflux? A randomised controlled trial. *J Vasc Surg* 2008; **48**: 173–178.

22. Gnat M, Mlineritsch B, Luschin-Ebengreth G *et al*. Adjuvant endocrine therapy plus zoledronic acid in premenopausal women with early-stage breast cancer: 5 year follow-up of the ABCST-12 bone mineral density substudy. *Lancet Oncol* 2008; **9**: 840–849.

23. Ruggiero R, Procaccini E, Piazza P *et al* Effectiveness of fibrin glue in conjunction with collagen patches to reduce seroma formation after axillary lymphadenectomy for breast cancer. *Am J Surg* 2008; **196**: 170–174.

Index

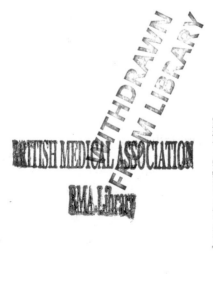